Carb Cycling

Special Edition – Two Books

The Ultimate Carb Cycling Fat Burning System With Quick Meal Plans

Josh Falenski

Carb Cycling Special Edition

The Ultimate Carb Cycling Fat Burning System With Quick Meal Plans

Published By:

*Dana Publishing
12804 Chillicothe Road #202
Chesterland, OH 44026*

Table of Contents

Conclusions...170

Carb Cycling

A Rapid Fat Loss Strategy That Actually Works and Keeps You Happy and Healthy

Includes Delicious and Simple Recipes

By Josh Falenski

Introduction to Carb Cycling

Starting a brand-new diet carries daunting obstacles that can serve to dissuade you from fully committing yourself. What's more, you may have tried a certain dietary plan before only to find that it was very difficult to maintain given your busy personal and professional life.

However, carb cycling is not a diet. In fact, it is merely a process through which you can increase and decrease your carb intake on a periodic cycle. This text will provide you will a bevy of meal plans and strategies to ensure that you reach your goals after implementing carb cycling into your dietary routine.

Moreover, you will find also find valuable information pertaining to the science behind carb cycling and carbohydrates for your body overall. This will give you a broader understanding of how carbs affect your body and the best ways to manipulate your carb intake for the better. As such, common misconceptions related to carb intake and the myths that dissuade people from consuming carbs will be extinguished entirely.

With experts and nutritional researchers currently working frantically to uncover the latest information and data related to cycling carbs, there is currently enough information to feel safe about adopting this dietary approach into your daily routine. As a result, you can begin to reap the benefits of cycling curbs immediately. However, this text will lay out some of the current grey areas and minor concerns expressed by nutrition experts with regard to carb cycling to that readers are given a wholly objective view and understanding about this dietary approach.

While all of our bodies are different on some level, there are shared characteristics with regard to the effects that an all-meat diet will have on us. Whether you are striving to build more muscle, increase strength, lose weight, boots total energy levels, endurance and enhance overall performance, this text provides all of the abundant information needed to reach your goals and get the most out of carb cycling. Notably, getting started with any new dietary routine can be rather difficult, this is why this book provides detailed strategies for how to implement carb cycling initially and provides diet plans to assist with this transition. As a result, readers will be ready to tack any and all challenges pertaining to carb cycling and will be able to reap the rewards of this routine for a prolonged period of time.

Where your health is concerned, there are no shortcuts and flash diets to help you reach your goals. If you are looking for prolonged dietary success, with results that last a lifetime, this book is by far the very best option to ensure that you maximize your full health potential and live your best life.

So, let's get started.

Carb Cycling

Nutrition always comes in cycles. Initially, we were all told that we should refrain from eating excess fat. Thereafter, this cycle began to shift steadily, and we began chastising carbohydrates.

Indeed, at some level, fearing carbohydrates is warranted. Carbs comprise much of our calories on a daily basis. Moreover, consuming simple carbs found on candy, donuts and white bread, to name only a few, can trigger many adverse health effects— especially for those striving to shed weight or boost their overall health.

So, what do many people resort to? They end up deciding to just eliminate carbohydrates altogether. However, this type of extreme carb restriction is entirely unnecessary. On the other hand, consuming complex carbs— more leisurely known as the "good carbs"— will give your body appropriate fuel that it needs to make it through all of your intense workouts, but your day as a whole. This is precisely why cycling your carbs is an excellent strategy. In practice, all this means is that you will have to alternate low and high-carbohydrate days.

Implementing carb cycling, the practice of eating an elevated amount of carbs one particular day, only to be followed by a day with low carb consumption, has proven benefits across many spectrums of physical fitness. So, whether you are a high-level athlete or someone who has only minimal physical activity, this dietary approach can benefit you immensely. This diet requires that you switch between high and low carb consumption during the week. The logic that undergirds this diet is based on the diet that you garner all of the internet benefits of consuming high-carbs on days when you are the most physically active, and then alternate to low-carbs on those days where your activity is limited.

When your body is active, you will use up your storage of carbs for extra energy. In this way, you days of highest carb consumption will be aligned with all of your days of training—these are the periods when our bodies can use that fuel the best. Indeed, this can carry great benefits for you. For example, the immersed in a high-intensity training session, your body will be fueled with enough carbs to help you push through the challenging physical demands of the workout. On the other hand, on days of recovery and rest, your cutting back on carbohydrates will reduce empty calories without carrying the ling being too limited for the remainder of the week.

Notably, there remains no amount for the number of carbohydrates that can be consumed on low or high-carb days. The amount that you consume hinges on the intensity and specific form of training that you are undergoing, along with the total amount of workout that you perform during the week.

Just like any diets, there is a bevy of ways to cycle your carb consumption that are available online. However, keep in mind that you must take into account what your specific needs are— this text will assist with that purpose.

Before you implement carb cycling, there are four key ideas that you should consider. As such, cycling carbs will require you to put together a detailed plan— more so than many other diets. This is because you will have to count grams for your meal plans, along with measuring and weighing them as well. Now, certain applications are available that can certainly help you keep track of all of the components needed for carb cycling. If you prefer a diet that is a bit looser and offers a more flexible approach, you may find that cycling carbs will be far too stringent for you. For those who are okay with, or even prefer guidelines, there are four key ideas that you should keep in mind:

1. Be Aware of the Specific Number of Calories That Your Body Requires

Put together a specific goal for your calorie intake. This goal should be something that you strive for everyday. For instance, if you wish to shed weight, start by taking your body weight and multiply it by 10x. This is the number of calories that you should aim for each and every day. If you want to maintain your weight, x by 12; if you wish to gain weight, x by 15.

2. Be Sure to Be Balanced with Macros

Divide these calories amongst all of your macronutrients—these include fat, protein, and carbohydrates. Moreover, proteins and carbohydrates offer 4 cals./gram. On the other hand, fat will give you around 9 cals./gram.

Additionally, along with cycling carbs, you should strive for around 1.5grams of protein/pound per each pound of your body weight. You should compensate for the rest with fats that are healthy. Moreover, on days of high-carbohydrate consumption, you are required to raise the calorie and carbs that you intake, all the while maintaining the fat and protein consumption stable.

3. Make Sure That You Do Not Forget to Consume Fiber

Whenever you consume a fewer amount of carbs, keep in mind to maintain your consumption of fiber. Indeed, days of lower carbohydrate consumption should not exclude healthy, fiber-rich foods such as apples and or broccoli. Your focus needs to be centered on eliminating sugar and other simple carbohydrates-rich foods.

Load up on fiber and nutrient-rich vegetables, fruit, beans, oats, quinoa, and other quality grains.

4. Make Sure That You Are Consuming A Sufficient Amount of Food— Even on Those Days of Low-Carb Intake

Our brains operate on carbohydrates— glucose, to be more specific. If there is not any immediately accessible glucose, your body will use other sources such as protein— this is disastrous for those striving to maintain and add more lean muscle onto your frame. This is precisely the reasoning that drives the notion of consuming over 140 grams of carbohydrates on days of low-carb intake. This ensures that you do not spend your day in a lazy, unproductive haze all day long.

Chapter 1
The Basics of Carb Cycling

With many studies conducted on this topic, and lingering debates surrounding the notion of carbohydrate intake, this book is intended to delve deeply into how cycling carb intake carries many benefits for reducing fat percentage, specifically. While cutting down the percentage of fat on your body is subject to many different factors, with some being pre-existing- such as genetics- this text will explain how cycling carb intake is the most reliable and consistent methods of reducing one's overall body fat.

Granted, starting a new diet is a very challenging process and carries many obstacles mentally, physically and even emotionally. However, by systematically approaching your diet, with careful consideration given to how your body is responding to the new changes that you are implementing, you will be well on your way to enjoying all of the inherent benefits that carb cycling has to offer you.

While there are certainly numerous benefits associated with your intake of carbs, it is integral to note that *more* medical research still needs to be done in order to unveil all of the effects and potential benefits associated with this process. Given the number of studies of dependable studies that have already been conducted, along with the plethora personal testimonies and anecdotes from dependable sources, you do not have to worry much about how this diet will affect you. The need for more research is merely a manner through which more information can be uncovered pertaining to cycling one's carb consumption. This will provide you with a much deeper understanding of the specific ways that this diet will influence your body and help you reach your desired goals.

What Are Carbohydrates?

Carbs are present in nature and we commonly employ them within our bodies to house disperse and house energy. From a scientific perspective, carbs are molecules that are comprised of hydrogen, oxygen and carbon. Moreover, carbs include starches and sugar that are in fruit, dairy and also many grains. Broken down within our body's natural digestive systems, these carbs are then broken into simple sugars known as glucose, before being wholly absorbed directly through the intestines. Thereafter, these sugars enter our bloodstream providing energy for our brains along with fuel for all of our muscles.

All of the energy and focus required for keeping track of your carb intake and meal planning might have very likely inhibited you from posting a certain question: What exactly is a carbohydrate? All the foods that you consume are made up of a particular combination of protein, carbs and fats that are directly converted by your body into sources of raw materials needed for life and or fuel for your daily life. As they are excellent for offering energy rather quickly, learning how to manage them is integral to understanding ailments such as diabetes because carbs are broken and converted into glucose. As such, glucose is the sugar that those suffering from diabetes carry in excess within their respective bloodstreams.

The main three components of all carbs- oxygen, carbon and hydrogen- can all be conjoined together and thus serve many different purposes. Also, it is important to note that your body is able to retrieve carbs from food as well as from its own processes of making carbs. In the same way that plants are able to create starch to store their natural glucose, humans carry their own glucose unit knows as glycogen- also commonly referred to as animal starch. Once glucose enters into your bloodstream following a meal, your body's cells gather the available glucose so that it can be employed for energy or in a manner that packages molecules of glycogen however your body needs.

Very little glycogen is found within the foods that we humans consume. This is precisely because the glycogen is broken down after the slaughtering of an animal. Accordingly, this is why meat isn't a source of carbs. Thankfully, your body is able to hold extra glycogen to control against low and high glucose in your blood. When the glucose levels in your blood fall, such as while we are asleep, your liver will use these extra glycogen reserves to deliver glycogen to your bloodstream, thereby maintaining glycogen levels at just the right levels to ensure that our brains and bodies are sufficiently fueled.

When we are undergoing prolonged periods of exercise or fasting, the amount of glycogen made from sources of food that you consume can run dry; however, your liver is uniquely able to make more glucose from scratch, thereby ensuring that your body's glucose levels are maintained at sufficient levels. Once the amount of glucose in your blood reaches levels that are too high, a hormone that signals that your body is well fed, known as insulting, informs the liver to refrain from delivering glucose to your blood.

Intake has been a very popular topic for many, many years. Even more, many diets that have been adopted and successfully implemented by people in recent years often entirely exclude carbs. Though macronutrients are not inherently harmful to your health, intaking carbs most be uniquely adjusted to each individual so that they garner the very best results. As a result, many people have recently started to cycle their carb intake to retrieve results and maximize their chances of reaching all of their dietary goals. Indeed, this has now become widely known as carb cycling.

This approach is used on a common basis to drop body fat, sustaining maximum and peak physical performance, or even use through a plateau of weight loss. The ways in which people uniquely implement carb cycling is tailored to their individual schedules, health history and commitment to exercising. As such, some people will alter their intake of carbs on a day-to-day basis, and other people will implement carb cycling for more prolonged periods of time with low, moderate as well as high-carbohydrate diets. In other words, cycling your carbohydrate intake is targeted to time carb intake to periods when it will provide the most benefit while excluding carbohydrates when they are no longer needed and will not provide the best results.

Overall, cycling carbohydrates strives to effectively gauge your carb intake to periods of peak benefit for your body. Also, carb cycling will limit, and even exclude altogether, carbs when your body no longer needs them.

<u>You are able to effectively strategize your carb consumption using certain factors:</u>

- Body Composition: Many people will cut carbs during their diet, only to reintegrate carbs during periods of muscle building or performance periods.

- Rest Days and Training: One popular method is more intake of carbs on days of training and less intake of carbohydrates during rest periods.

- Refeed Schedules: Another effective approach is implementing 1 or more days at high-carbohydrate consumption to perform "refeed" during an extended diet.

- Special Competitions or Events: Athletes often consume carbs at a high rate before a specific event

- Form of Training: People often tailor their intake of carbs depending on the overall period of particular exercising sessions.

- Levels of Body Fat: Many people will cycle carbs based on the body fat levels that these people carry.

A typical week of cycling one's carbohydrates will often incorporate two ways of high-carb intake, along with two days of moderate carbohydrate consumption and then 3 days of low-carb consumption.

Also, the intake of protein is typically the same between these days of carb cycling. However the intake of fat will tend to vary depending on the intake of carbs. Usually, days of high carbohydrate consumption will mean lower-fat intake, whereas days low-carb intake will be high in fat. Cycling carbohydrates is a strategy of dieting that is advanced and will need enhanced manipulation and programming compared to a usual diet. As a brief capitulation, the process of carb cycling is a dieting approach that is specific to altering one's consumption of carbs based on certain factors.

While carbs provide energy — we need them to perform at an optimal level — we don't need carbs all the time. That's why it makes sense to use them only when needed the most — during intense physical training. On the days we're not training to our fullest — maybe it's an off day or a light training day — cut back on carbs to help improve metabolic flexibility and help the body learn to use fat as fuel. And because the body uses stored glycogen (sugar from carbs) during training, strategic high-carb days can help replenish your supply and increase strength during workouts.

The other cool thing about carb cycling is that targeting your carb intake around training days can help improve insulin sensitivity. If you're insulin sensitive, the body only needs to release a small amount of insulin to use and store glucose (blood sugar). This factor alone can keep you from putting on too much body fat and prevent you from getting Type 2 diabetes.

To get even better weight-loss results, pair carb cycling with a caloric deficit (reduce calorie intake and/or burn more calories).

Your Four-Week Carb-Cycling Meal Plan

While there are a handful of ways to interpret carb cycling, this plan is based around your training routine. Our plan is laid out for you to use the high-carb and moderate-to-low-fat and protein menus for endurance/cardio or intense training days. On off days and weight-training days, you'll follow the high-protein, high-fat and low-carb menus. If you're someone who doesn't do any cardio or does cardio and weights on the same day, use the high-carb days on weight-training days and follow the low-carb days on off days.

Since we're changing the number of carbs we're eating based on training, we're going to do the same with protein and fats.

You'll notice that on high-carb days, protein and fat are reduced, while on low-carb days, you'll be eating more protein and fat throughout the day to maintain satiety and keep calories similar throughout the week.

Though protein has been lowered on high-carb days, it's still considered "high" in the mainstream nutrition world. This is because no matter what day it is — training, endurance or off day — protein is always important. It helps boost metabolism, burn fat, improve recovery and build/maintain muscle. Plus, it helps keep us full and satisfied long after eating.

Here is how to adjust your meal plan so that it comfortably fits with your unique routine.

The meal plan is laid out as follows:

Mondays, Wednesdays and Fridays should have weight-training with low-carbohydrate intake

Sundays will be an off-day with low-carb intake

Tuesdays, Thursdays and Saturdays will be a cardiovascular training day for endurance— with high-carb intakes.

This calendar is to be followed on a skip-a-day approach to its cardio and specific training days. If you find that you prefer a routine for your workouts that are more than two days, with one day off approach, all you really have to do is employ the days for the endurance meal-plan for the training days, and the day-off menu for the rest days.

With carb cycling, you are certainly able to adjust your unique meal plan in a manner that is derived from your unique schedule. This means that if you work long hours with very little time to workout or remain active, you can manipulate your diet in a specific way that allows you to maintain healthy eating and cycling of your carbohydrates.

Also, once you adjust your diet plan according to your unique schedule and find that you have yet to fully experience results that you had expected, you should try cutting your carbohydrate consumption to only 30g/day on your *days off*. Keep in mind that these are only days where you are resting and do not have intense training.

Salmon Poke Bowl

This recipe makes 2 servings and requires approximately 30 mins of preparation.

The serving size is 1 Salmon Poke Bowl; it contains:

- **549 Total Calories**
- **39g Fat**
- **370 mg. Sodium**
- **32g Carbs**
- **6g Fiber**
- **4g Sugar**

What's in It

- Salmon (3oz.)
- Cabbage (cubed to 3/4 dices)
- Chives (1 T)
- Cucumber (1/4 cup)
- Sesame seeds (1 T)

How's it Made

1. Add rice to a medium sized bowl
2. In a medium-sized bowl, whisk together all ingredients.

3. Add Salmon

4. Now, garnish the bowl with the chives that have been chopped, along with the sesame seeds

<u>Pizza Mac n' Cheese Casserole</u>

This recipe will make 6 servings and will require approximately 60 minutes if preparation.

<u>It contains:</u>

- **360 Total Calories**
- **3g Saturated Fat**
- **21g. Protein**
- **58g carbs**

<u>What's in It</u>

- Whole Wheat Elbow (2 cups)
- Gluten-free elbow or noodles
- noodles
- non-fat milk (1/2 cup)
- Cornstarch (1 T)
- Mozzarella Cheese (1/4 cup of partly skimmed + 1 cup)
- Butter (1 T)
- Turkey Pepperonis (12)
- Tomato Sauce (1/2 cup)
- Onion Powder
- Garlic Powder

<u>How's it Made</u>

1. Prepare noodles just as the package indicates until it reaches al dente.

2. In a saucepan, throw in the 1/2 cup of non-fat milk, Salt (1/4 teaspoon), Oregano (1/4 teaspoon), garlic powder (1/4 teaspoon), Onion powder (1/4 teaspoon). Next, simmer.

3. In another bowl, stir the cornstarch along with the non-fat milk (1/4 cup), add this to the saucepan from step 2.

4. Mix together. Keep stirring directly over the heat until the sauce has become thick. Continue doing this for about 5 mins.

5. Keep stirring this until it has completely melted all the way through — next, butter into a saucepan (1 tablespoon).

6. Mix with the noodles that you have cooked along with the cheese until it has been combined. Add this mixture of cheese and noodles to the mixed casserole dish.

7. Pour the tomato sauce directly over the top of the dish. Add Mozzarella cheese topped with turkey pepperonis (12 pieces).

8. Bake @ 375 degrees for 30 mins.

Pesto Chicken Sandwich

This recipe will make only 1 serving and will require 30 minutes of preparation.

It Contains:

- **425 Calories**
- **26g Fat**
- **6g Fat**
- **32g Protein**
- **580 mg Sodium**
- **26g Carbs**
- **7g Fiber**
- **6g Sugar**
-

What's in It

- Whole Wheat Bread (2 slices)
- Grilled Chicken Breast (4oz)
- Pesto Sauce (1 T)
- Mozzarella Cheese (1 Slice)
- Tomato (3 slices)
- Olive Oil Mayo (1-3 T)

<u>How's it Made</u>

1. Warm the skillet over low to medium heat. You can also use an indoor grill if one is easily accessible to you.

2. Put olive oil mayo only onto one side of each slice of bread. Then, apply the pesto directly on the other side of each slice of bread.

3. Start to put together the sandwich by beginning with the chicken, followed by tomato and finally end with a piece of mozzarella.

4. Apply the top of the sandwich with the second slice of bread and then put into the warmed skillet or your indoor grill.

5. Now, cook for around 2 min on each side, if you are using a skillet. Conversely, you can cook for however long until the bread has been completely toasted and all of the mozzarella has been melted if using an indoor grill.

*** It is entirely up to you if you want to use a skillet or an indoor grill.*

French Toast Including Bananas (Caramelized)

This recipe will make 1 serving and will require approximately 30 minutes of preparation.

It Contains:

- **500 Total Calories**
- **28g Fat**
- **33g Carbs**
- **27g Protein**
- **10g Sugar**

What's in It

- Large eggs (1)
- Egg White (1)
- Cinnamon (Just a dash)
- Nutmeg (Just a dash)
- Vanilla Extract (2 Tablespoons)
- Whole-Wheat Bread (3 slices)
- Butter (2.5 Tablespoons of butter)
- Banana (Medium size; slice into 1/4 rounds)
- Maple Syrup (1 Tablespoon)
- Vanilla Extract (1/4 Teaspoon)

<u>How's it Made</u>

1. In one small bowl, whip the following together: cinnamon, egg, egg white, nutmeg and vanilla

2. Coat and then dip all slices of bread into the mixture from step 1. C Then, cook right on the grill until it appears to be brown or golden brown. Cook for only 1 min. on each side.

3. Place over medium heat after you add butter. After this butter has melted, throw in cinnamon, banana, maple syrup and vanilla extract. Then, stir so that you combine until fully cooked. Do this for about 3 minutes.

4. Lastly, pour the bananas on the French toast. Add whipped cream or cinnamon if you wish.

As elaborated upon earlier in this text, cycling carbohydrates carries the ability to offer many benefits that alternative diets simply cannot provide. By having stages of high and low-carbohydrate intake, you will likely garner any of the same benefits that the other diets can offer, devoid of some of the negative components of these diets.

Some of the very best benefits of diets that are low in carb intake will provide better sensitivity to insulin, more turning of fat, enhanced metabolic health and even improvements in cholesterol.

Refeeds of high-carbs carry many positive benefits on hormones while on a diet, which also includes some thyroid hormones and leptin. Also, these factors will play a vital role with regard to prolonged success in dieting because hormones also play an integral role in metabolism, performance in exercise and hunger.

Should You Have Cheat Days?

Also, there are certainly some carbs that one should be sure to avoid, with the exception of certain special circumstances and events such as Christmas, birthdays and other situations. These occasions should be fully enjoyed so that you are giving your mind and body a break and opportunity to recharge. Numerous studies have shown the value of dieting breaks for refueling your mind and body, allowing you to come back to your dietary routine stronger than ever before. Be sure to take advantage of this opportunity should you feel that you could use a break from your diet.

Carbohydrate cycling is a very beneficial approach to those who are striving to make the most of their diet, health and performance for exercising.

The unique individual mechanisms that undergird cycling carbs are very strongly backed up by in-depth and peer-reviewed research from the medical and nutrition communities. However, there is still no research that has been conducted on the topic of the effects that a prolonged carb cycling diet has on our bodies and cellular function.

As opposed to high or low-carb diets that are chronic, a calm balance between the two can be very beneficial for people from a psychological and even physical standpoint. If implementing carb cycling for losing fat from your body, make sure that your intake of protein is sufficient and that you are able to sustain a calorie deficit. Be sure to always temper and experiment with protocol and amount of carbs that you consume so that you find the very best fit for that approach that works best for you.

Variation and Manipulation

If people put together a plan to consume more carbs at regular intervals, their bodies will not get closer to reaching the coveted starvation phase. Not to mention, these people will still be able to lose weight and drop their body fat percentage if they manage to consume less overall calorie than they spend.

Days of higher carb consumption will boost thyroid output and manage the hunger that people feel. Alerting the consumption of carbs will also assist with people taking full advantage of particular anabolic hormones, such as insulin.

Some important facets of carbohydrate cycling:

There are numerous approaches and strategies for cycling carbohydrates. Nonetheless, the common thread that tethers them together is the not in that fat and protein consumption remain relatively stable and consistent while carb intake is being manipulated.

Cycling carbs also usually incorporates cycling calories. Because carbs carry less than 5 calories per gram, altering carb intake when trying to keep protein and fat can play an integral role in altering calorie intake. On days where carbs— typically calories— are boosted are typically known as "re-feed" days.

Those people who are interested in boosting their muscle mass require a surplus of calories. However, if these people consume too many calories for prolonged periods of time, they are likely to gain too much body fat. Therefore, one strategically effective approach to boosting gaining muscle instead of fat during a phase of muscle gaining is through cycling carbs. The menus while on this diet are put together with the intention of keeping your weekly schedule in mind so that you are able to create a calorie surplus on an ephemeral basis, rather than a prolonged of time that will raise your overall body fat content. In addition, this will aid strength and gains of lean mass.

Here are some other tips that you may find helpful with regard to implementing and sustaining the results of carb cycling:

- Structure the diet routine with basic calorie requirements and levels of activity as the foundation.
- Choose the re-feed days ahead of time so that you are prepared and not caught up in a fluster— this will evidently lead to poor decisions.
- On days of re-feeding, your body will continue to accept carbs the best immediately in the morning, as wells during periods of high-physical exercise.

Overall, there are a few things that you should keep in mind as it pertains to cycling your carb intake:

- After choosing on a specific routine for cycling your carbs, you must then establish your goal for consuming calories.
- Second, set a specific and manageable goal for your protein consumption. The main key here is that this goal be *manageable* insofar as it does not conflict with any of your already established dietary goals.
- Third, fat an intake mark for your consumption of fat. Be sure to keep in mind that this goal be fairly consistent.

- Lastly, choose a carb consumption target for the days of the diet.

Chapter 2
Carb Cycling for Athletes

For any serious athlete, or anyone who exercises on a regular basis, maximizing your energy levels is incredibly important. This is especially critical if you also have a demanding career and need to balance your work life with your exercise and family life. With all of these moving parts and seemingly unending train of demands, it is integral that your diet is able to afford you with enough energy to keep up with your life at every stage.

Indeed, fueling your body is paramount for maximizing your body's ability to perform at its peak capacity. Carb cycling ensures that your path to reaching your goals and getting the absolute most out of your body is made easier and is done in the healthiest manner possible. Indeed, dieting in the healthiest way possible should always be your goal. If you choose another route, perhaps one that seems as though it is an easy shortcut to success, you will likely fail to see the best results and are more likely to plateau due to the diet itself being poorly laid out and formulated— either by you or whoever developed the diet.

Prior to delving deeply into how carb cycling benefits athletes, it is important to first note the different ways that athletes benefit from carbs. This will provide you with a greater breadth of knowledge and a deeper understanding of the layered benefits and effects that carbs carry for an athlete's body and performance.

Moreover, numerous sports nutrition experts have criticized that typical and rudimentary rules of feeding are no longer considered in the west to uncover the next new strategy for dieting— one that surpasses all of the other regimens and eventually creates the path to enhanced and maximized peak performance.

Due to the general misconception about limiting the overall intake of carbs for reasons related to health in the physically inactive population becoming more prevalent, many of forgotten that many top athletes have a need for consuming foods that are high in carbs to enhance the storage of muscle glycogen, while also delivering carbs to muscles in the midst of demanding training and exercise.

Carbs Are Still King for Training at High-Intensity

Despite the bevy of brand-new data that has been produced in recent years and a continually evolving awareness about how athletes manage to metabolize food, nutrition experts overwhelmingly agree that the main facets of sports nutrition have yet to change very much over the past 20 years or so.

While these nutrition experts certainly acknowledge that research suggests that an athlete's requirement for protein and fat is much higher today than in previous eras, one component that remains evident currently as ever is an athlete need to replenish their bodies with carbs following a hard training session or competition. Indeed, carbs are an essential component of sustaining an athlete's body, performance and overall health.

While dietary protein and certain fats offer the needed energy in order to perform physical activity, carbs are quite easily the most efficient metabolized substrate in our bodies and they are also the one y macronutrients that are able to be broken down fast enough to provide more energy and strength in the midst of training. In this way, those fast-twitch muscle fibers are constantly replenished and infused with sufficient nutrients to sustain performance and maximum energy levels.

Further. Many nutrition experts will point to statistics and new and updated data that many athletes consistently fail to eat sufficient amounts of carbs to completely replenish their bodies— specifically their reserves of muscle glycogen. A failure to do so leads to performance decrements, especially when intense training is consistently implemented on a regular basis.

Slowly Absorbed Versus Rapidly Absorbed Carbohydrates

Nutrition experts and researchers claim that during intense exercise, and even beforehand, the rate at which a carb enters into the bloodstream can directly impact the intensity of the training as well as the overall duration of the training as well. This is significant because it highlights that the rate that our bodies absorb carbs and reap the benefits of replenishing can be manipulated and should be taken into consideration.

Additionally, high-carb beverages and foods that are absorbed rapidly are preferred for giving our muscles energy before and during intense training and performance.

In recent years, many nutrition experts for sports alleged GI (glycemic index) carb levels that were on the lower side and show-up in our bloodstream at a slower rate, might very well be preferred prior to exercising simply because they manage the appearance of glucose in our bloodstreams. Nevertheless, this assumption by nutrition researchers has yet to be supported by data— experts still point to new research that suggests that there is no difference between pre-event consumption of foods that are low in GI.

In the immediate hours following intense training, new research suggests that foods that are high in carbs and nutritious are able to effectively alter the hormonal milieu responsible for speeding the process of glycogen resynthesis in our bloodstreams.

Low-Carbohydrate Diets for Athletic Performance

With a bevy of supportive analytics and data for the importance of carbs within the diet of an athlete, many nutritional experts profess a lot of concern pertaining to the growing popularity amongst individuals that are very active on a regular basis.

Many training and dieting routines such as the well-known "training-low" approach, which is a specific form of nutrition that is per iodized, has been around for just over a decade.

These types of nutritional approach are indicative of low-carb nutrition for purposes of performance. Accordingly, nutrition experts claim that these types of approaches are mostly fads as opposed to carrying any practical benefit.

Drawing on the current data available, nutritional experts consistently question and critique the inherent value provided by consuming low-carb diets. Also, they question the value of diets that promote ketones for enhancing one's performance. While research from the past claims that people who are more physically active are far more capable of adapting to using ketone bodies as sources of fuel when trying to operate on low to moderate levels of carbs. What's more is these individuals might even be more capable of conserving carbs and burning fat during training at low-intensity.

Moreover, nutritional experts claim that the prolonged use of these types of eating routines can be harmful to an athlete's overall performance. Many nutritional experts had even claimed that these diets could also negatively affect one's mood, cognitive capacities, levels of fatigue, as well as an inability to remain focused on their tasks. These symptoms are cited by nutritional experts as reasons for staying away from low-carb diet routines.

Other experts cite data pertaining to a low-carb diet's ability to damage skeletal muscles during exercise and or competition.

Indeed, low-carb storages in one's body carry sprawling effects in many different areas pertaining to their health, athletic performance and mood. Not to mention, many nutritional experts and nutrition researchers have referenced data suggesting that as the dehydration levels of athletes increases during training, they tend to rely more on the carb storages within their bodies for increases in energy. This gives credence to the claim that additional stores of carbs within one's body carry many benefits.

On the whole, most nutrition experts claim that low-carbohydrate stores make it difficult to sustain the intensity levels at which most competitive and serious recreational athletes train and compete.

As our understanding of the needs that athletes have from a nutritional perspective has increased abundantly recently along with the tools through which we measure how we metabolize food, the main components of sports nutrition have remained unchanged over the last 20 years or so.

While it is mainly understood that an athlete's requirement for protein is slightly higher than previously thought, one remaining factor that is true today as it has been for years is the notion that an athlete's need for carbs is an integral factor of a diet. Although fat and protein are very capable of offering the needed energy in order to perform physical exercise, carbs are the only macronutrient that is able to be broken down at a sufficient pace to offer energy during the periods of intense training.

Despite these realities, there still remains the need for additional study in order to uncover the full spectrum of effects and needs of those who are physically active on a regular basis in their daily lives.

The Role That Carbs Play for Most Athletes:

Carbs within our bodies offer a very important source of fuel for muscles and our brains while we are training or even exercising at a slow pace. Moreover, these carbs can be very easily manipulated through our diets and training— regardless of how intense these training sessions are.

A strongly advised strategy for promoting the best overall levels of performance during intense training or highly competitive competitions is adjusting the amount, timing and type of carbs— through beverage or food— in a manner that corresponds to the intensity of the session and what the athlete's body needs most.

Keeping a diet that is optimal for your health carries an abundant amount of positive results for athletes. Specifically, these include recovery, high-level performance, less chance of injury and maintaining an ideal weight and fat percentage. So, regardless of whether you are a high-level professional athlete, marginal athlete or an everyday person with little interest in exercise, managing your carb intake and properly cycling these carbs is integral to your overall health and how well your body performs in any endeavor you choose.

In one unique case, competitive elite race walkers were the subject of a study designed to measure and evaluate the effects of low-carb and high-fat diets in their performance.

This example carries considerable value with regard to measuring the specific and varied effects of carb consumption amongst elite athletes. Of course, most athletes are different, and the benefits and effects of nutrition on their bodies will vary according to their overall health, sport, injury history and genetics. Nevertheless, the research provides valuable information pertaining to the benefit of carbs for elite athletes in performance and training.

Days where you are consuming high levels of carbs, your metabolism will be boosted. Conversely, on days of low-carb consumption, the levels of insulin in your body will be just low enough that your body is able to burn fat while the amount of muscle that you have is maintained.

In this way, on days of low-carb consumption, our bodies tend to burn off fat rather than carbs. This combination lets your body burn off the maximum amount of fat while its muscle content is maintained. Remember, not all carbs are the same. Indeed, there are carbs that are good for your body such as complex carbs which trigger a more delayed change in the levels of glucose in your blood. Not to mention, there are cars that are bad for your body— these are simple carbs that raise the level of glucose in your blood. These are foods like candy, donuts and fries— these certainly do not have any role to play in your overall health and should, for the most part, be avoided. Namely, you should try to retrieve most or all of your carbohydrates from whole grains, veggies, whole oats, legumes and fruits.

Getting most or all of your veggies, in this way, will allow you to nourish your body with the best carbs and nutrients possible. Carrying this mentality into your carb cycling diet ensures that you maximize this diet so that you reach your goals and get the absolute most out of all of your dieting efforts.

Guidelines for Carb Cycling

1) Low carbohydrate consumption for off-days and days of rest

Carbs on this day should primarily come from green veggies. Do not worry about an exact number of carbs, as long as you are getting your carbohydrates from green veggies your intake will be low enough.

2) High carb intake on intense training days

Carbs on this day should come from complex carb sources primarily, but on this day, you can also add in some starchy carbs before and after your lifting session.

3) Alternate between high- and low-carb days

Never have two high-carb days in a row.

If you are unable to burn off that pesky body fat, or if every time you do your strength levels plummet, give carb cycling a try.

Next, let's delve into manipulating macronutrients to our advantage. Burning fat and building muscle is the name of the game so let's take a look at how each of these plays their unique role in the diet.

Protein intake will remain relatively unchanged throughout the diet. The only caveat would be to increase it slightly if gains are stalling. A good route to take is to go from 1 gram per pound of body weight to 1.25 grams. You can further increase this to 1.5 grams if you still feel you need to kick start your muscle-gaining efforts.

Fats will vary slightly relative to carb intake. Your baseline will be .25 grams per pound of bodyweight or roughly 20-30% of total daily calories. So, for our 200-pound individual example, he will need 50 grams per day as a baseline. On low carb days, you can increase healthy fats by 50% to curtail any loss of energy and to preserve hormone function for those intense workouts.

Carbohydrate will be the most manipulated macronutrient on this diet plan. You will have low, medium and high carb days depending on the number of training days and intensity levels.

A medium day will consist of intake of 1.5 grams per pound of bodyweight and they will fall on regular training days for the upper body. High carb days will take you to 2.25 grams per pound of bodyweight and be reserved for high-intensity workouts such as a heavy leg day or a prolonged and intense bout of weight training such as a full body routine or extra HIIT training.

The low days will force your body to tap into its fat stores for energy. After a length of time, your metabolism will start taking a hit and need a few extra calories to rev back up. Medium and high days are installed to help refuel glycogen stores and get the furnace burning once again and help support muscle gain.

Here is an outline for an individual that is 200 pounds:

200 pounds:
- Low-carbohydrate day: 110 grams
- Medium-carbohydrate day: 310 grams
- High-carbohydrate day: 460 grams
- If fat loss is stalling after a few weeks, add a few more low and/or medium carb days.
- On low carb days, don't forget to increase healthy fats – but just slightly.
- If you feel muscle gains are plateauing, increase protein to 1.25 and then 1.5 later on.
- If you have sensitivity toward carbs, limit your high carb day to one day per week and increase fats.

Muscle building, fat torching sample diet plan (amounts are approximated for a 200-pound individual)

3 tips that many athletes make when cycling their carbs:

Mistake #1: You focus on carbs and ignore the other macros.

Carb cycling is something of a misnomer—it's not just about carbs. Sometimes, people reduce their carb intake on low-activity days but eat more fat and protein on those days, so much that they're getting the same number of calories overall. If that happens, you're not going to see much fat loss in the long run. When carbs fluctuate, your total calorie intake should, too.

Cycle fix: Find your maintenance calories, the number that keeps you at your current weight, with an online calculator.

On easy days, get 10 to 20 percent less of your calories from carbs without upping your fat or protein intake. Keep in mind that there are four calories per gram of carb, so if you eat 2,000 calories per day, reduce your carb intake by 50 grams (roughly 200 calories worth) on days you're not training heavily.

Mistake #2: Your calorie intake varies way too much.

The 10-to-20-percent rule applies specifically to carbs, but there should never consistently be more than a 33 percent difference in the total number of calories you eat from one day to the next. That type of variance can hurt the recovery and make it harder for you to stick to a carb cycling plan, says Zach Moore, CSCS, a Bloomington, Indiana-based nutrition coach at Precision Nutrition.

Cycle fix: Eat at least 68 percent of your typical energy intake on reduced-carb days, Moore says. That means at least 1,360 calories for people who typically eat 2,000 per day.

Mistake #3: You treat high-carb days as cheat days.
People often use high-output days as excuses to eat whatever they want, Moore says. That's a flawed plan because it's easy for unhealthy habits to become more regular.

Cycle fix: Indulgences are fine now and then, but your main focus should be on nutrient-dense options, Moore says. Aim for whole foods, like potatoes and oats on high-carb days and eggs and nuts on low-carb days.

Chapter 3

Losing Weight and
the Science Behind Carb Cycling

The Science of Cycling Carbs

As a new diet, this diet is somewhat developed from the factors that undergird manipulating carbs. As such, there are still not many substantiated and controlled studies that directly investigate a carb cycling routine. In basic terms, carb cycling is a mechanism through which we try to match our body's requirement for glucose or calories.

Theoretically, this method will certainly maximize the overall benefits that carbs offer our bodies. As explained in the earlier part of this text, the benefits that carbs give our bodies is immense. While the factors that support cycling carbs certainly support its implementation, it should be viewed with some caution due to a lack of direct research about its complete effect on our health. However, this is mainly pertinent for individuals that have a history of medical concerns, especially those that have had concerns and issues related to diets that they have implemented.

The science of carb cycling converges with math, but it's rather simple math at that. On high-carb days, try to eat between 1 and 1.5 grams of carbs for every pound of your total body weight. Or make it simpler yet and set your "high-carb limit" at 200 grams on high-carb days. On low-carb days, cut this number in half. (Just remember to count only those starchy carbs; fruits and vegetables are low in carbs as well as calories and should be excluded from your "carb count.")

Here are some important things that you should keep in mind before fully implementing the carb-cycling diet into your routine for any period of time:

1. Days of High-Carb Consumption Are to Be Implemented on Intense Training Days:

Perhaps the most important thing that you should be aware of as it pertains to this to carb cycling is that you should put your highest carb consumption on days where you plan on having your most intense workout sessions. So, for instance, this means that you should be eating the most carbs on heavy workout days, or on days that involve a full body workout. This is because our bodies require carbohydrates at our most intense levels on these specific times of the week. Moreover, consuming these prior to exercising will give your body enough fuel so that you have enough energy to push your way through the most challenging aspects of the workout. Thereafter, having carbs right after the workout will help replenish and nourish your body so that you recover fast and that your body has enough energy to have another intense workout the next day or later in the week. Specifically, this is also great for building more muscle as it will allow you to lift more weight for longer periods of time.

Because you want your carb consumption to be put to the best use possible in a manner that allows you to maximize results, along with preventing them from being converted into body fat, you have to ensure that you are timing them correctly throughout the course of the week. Planning your carb cycling, in this way, is an integral part of making sure that this method works best for you. Coupled with already having knowledge about how your body works and strategies work best for training and exercising your body, planning your intake of carbs in a strategic manner is key to getting the absolute most out of your body while training or, more generally, in your everyday life.

2. You May Gain Water Weight

You should also be aware of, and prepare for, possibly gaining a little bit of weight at times of implementing the high-carb day. With every carb that is consumed, your body will then hold on to 4g of water. So, when consuming 250- 350g of carbs on days high-carb intake, this will tend to add up extremely quickly.

For people whose body composition is already leaner, they will experience this effect mostly due to water weight simply being more noticeable on their leaner body. Not to worry, this is a completely normal process and is very common. And, thankfully, this excess water weight does not signal that your body is gaining fat. <u>This water weight gain will certainly recede within a few days on the normal low-carb intake regimen</u>.

Now, it is important to be aware of whether you are someone who struggles with weight gain from a psychological perspective. If this is you, then perhaps cycling carbs is dangerous for you and you should reconsider. Indeed, temporary water weight gain tends to common accompany this dietary routine. Moreover, be prepared for this to possibly take place prior to undertaking the diet.

3. Select Carbs That Are Highest in Complex Carbohydrates or Glucose

As it pertains to selecting which food to consume when undertaking a carb cycling regimen for losing fat, you need to consider glucose. This include either sources of simple glucose (which should be consumed somewhere near the workout period where they will incidentally be absorbed much faster) or complex carbs that will be broken into glucose by your body naturally.

What should be avoided in this instance is fructose (as in high-fructose corn syrup to be specific), because this form of carb will interact differently with your body and will not have any of the positive benefits that accompany glucose.

If, for example, you consume a lot of fructose during periods of high-carb consumption, there is a high likelihood that it will be turned into fat because it will not be stored within your muscles as quickly.

4. Lower Your Fat Consumption on High-Carb Days

Another integral consideration that you should keep in mind as you integrate a carb cycling regimen is that you need to decrease your fat intake on high-carb days. However, by lowering the overall fat intake, you will be allowing greater space for these carbs without consuming *too many* total calories.

In an ideal plan, you should try to stay within a 350-600 overall calorie limit on your days of low-carb intake in order to prevent the consumption of excess calories from being in a stalemate with your fat loss for that particular week.

5. Sustain Your Weekly Target Calorie Level for Losing Fat

As an appendage of the point above is that the overall week intake of calories should remain at a level that is needed for losing fat. For instance, when keeping your weight at 2300 calories per day, which is just slightly more than 15,400 per week, you will need to trigger an overall calorie deficit of 3500 calories per week or consume 11,900 total calories/week in order to shed one pound per week.

Standard diets require you to maintain a similar calorie level on every day of the week, this- requires you to consume 1700 calories/day. Now, consider whether you wanted to have 3 high-carb days to maximize the benefits and get the most results, you should set the calorie intake at 2400— just make sure that your weekly protein consumption remains consistent all week. As a result, because those 3 days equal nearly 7200 total calories, you will have 4700 calories that are remaining for the remaining 4 days, which is nearly 1100 calories for each.

You might be able to tell that these low carb days are very low in calories; however, following high-carb days, many people will find this to be rather easy and not too much of a struggle. If, for instance, you would rather not bring you low-carb days too low on the total amount of calorie that you consume, all you really have to do is bring the overall intake of calories on high-carb days lower. As a result, you will get more calories for low-carb days as well. This is significant because it demonstrates that you can certainly tinker and adjust your carb cycling in a manner that works best for you. This diet regimen is not overly stringent and strenuous insofar as it limits your capacity to play around with the math. Rather, you are able to adjust the calorie and carb levels to such a degree that you reap the most benefits without having to sacrifice comfort or put too much of a strain on your body and the way that you feel.

You can probably tell that the idea of carb cycling is really about balance. Finding ways to balance your intake of carbs and calories will enhance your overall enjoyment and the benefits that you enjoy from the diet. Just be sure that your weekly intake of carbs and calories is exactly where it needs to be and that you alter and adjust accordingly. After you establish your preferences, make sure that you start to distribute all of your calories thereafter.

Simple vs. complex carbs

With the only real standout being fibers, all carbs can be absorbed directly through one's intestines and then into their blood as sugar. Moreover, this then causes blood sugar levels to rise rather rapidly. Accordingly, this form of carb will determine if the blood sugar rise is stretched over a longer period or if it is more sudden.

Simple carbs, which you should try to avoid at all costs, are primarily found in cookies, ice cream and many products that are based in flour such as pasta and dairy products. Sugar that is found within these products, along with the white flours, is broken into glucose very quickly within the digestive system. This quick breaking down means an abundant amount of glucose is then wholly absorbed through our intestines and then flows directly into our bloodstream at one time. Consequently, this leads to a spike in our blood sugar. This rise in blood sugar within our bloodstream then triggers insulin to store the remaining energy as glycogen within our fat cells—otherwise referred to as fat gain.

On the other hand, complex carbs provide energy that we all require in order to sustain our nervous system and muscles functioning devoid of excess fat— or really any fat at all. This is simply because complex carbs, which are primarily found within whole grains such as starchy food (potatoes) as well as quinoa, will take a lot longer in order to convert into glucose within our digestive system. A more prolonged breaking down results in a very slow pace of absorption into our bloodstream. In this way, a longer absorption period will mean that there will be no rise in blood sugar, resulting in no activation of insulin; therefore, there will be zero storing of energy within the fat cells in our body.

So, with all of this being considered, you should not be afraid of eating carbs! Just be sure to consume only the complex ones, rather than the far more harmful simple ones. Foods that are full of sugar— mainly those that are prepared with white flour such as pasta— are the kinds that we tend to want to eat the most. These cravings can certainly be intense. Sadly, these carbs are most harmful to us and are the main cause of gaining weight. Indeed, there is also very little to no value from a nutritional standpoint in these foods.

In contrast, complex carbs are packed with vitamins that carry great value from a nutritional perspective for our bodies. In addition to this, complex carbs can assist with losing weight because you will feel more satisfied for a long period of time. This is due to the slower breaking down within our digestive system.

The specific factors that undergird cycling carbs indicate that it is very beneficial for losing weight and even lowering your overall levels of body fat. Technically, cycling carbs all assist with sustaining a certain level of physical performance all the while offering many of the same rewards as dietary regimens that are primarily low-carbs.

Just like pretty much any diet, the primary mechanism that supports losing weight are calorie deficits— such as consuming less than what your body is able to burn off over an extended period. Now, is a diet that involves cycling cards is adopted in concert with a calorie deficit you will begin to shed weight at a relatively fast pace. However, the complexity of this integrated approach is enough to trigger confusion amongst people who are new to dieting and thus dissuade them from carrying on with the diet.

On the other hand, many individuals would prefer carb cycling's inherent flexibility. Also, this may even improve performance and results for many people, thereby allowing them to experience long-term success as well. In short, cycling your carb intake will certainly help you lose weight provided you are able to maintain a calorie deficit. Consuming ample amounts of protein is also very useful.

Among the most predominate ideas behind cycling carbs is

setting a limit on carbs once your body does not require them. Moreover, carbohydrates can be used as fuel, in the same way as gas for your vehicle, to assist your cells with performing their functions.

Consuming a lot of carbs on certain days when you are not particularly active is fairly nonsensical due to your body needing less energy— in the same way that your vehicle does not need as much gas for a short ride through town compared to a prolong trip across the country.

In fact, carbohydrates that are not burned fully result in a surplus— this can inhibit the likelihood that you will lose weight, or even result in gaining weight. On the other hand, a limit of carbohydrates to 30 grams is quite low, even on days that are not particularly active as compared to other days. 30 grams is the total amount of carbs that are found within a cup of broccoli, an apple, as well as 4 small carrots. Instead, if you are looking for a better balance, you are well advised to employ what has become more widely known as "carb matching"— this is the practice of aligning your carbohydrate consumption with all of the energy requirements that your body has. Admittedly, these will certainly vary on any given day, or periods in the day.

Essentially, this method is aligned with consuming massive portions of whole carbs that are clean in order to provide more support during active hours during the day. Further, this also involves cutting your carb intake during periods of the day that are far less active. For a practical example, say you are planning to have a workout in the morning, you should eat oatmeal that is topped with some diced banana for your breakfast. However, if you are going to be in an office where you will be seated at a desk for an extended period of time, try having an avocado and veggies omelet with berries on the side. Also, as an alternative, a liquid morning diet is a great choice. Try having a protein scoop, along with some chia seed, hemp and frozen berries.

Complex carbs don't cause weight gain

A widely adopted misconception that many people tend to carry is that all carbs will cause you to gain weight and that by reducing carbs or cutting them out of your routine entirely, will boost your overall health. To fully grasp how and why this idea is flawed, you must first understand the intricate and complex ways that our bodies tend to interact with carbs— and what is the actual cause of gaining more fat onto your body.

Indeed, all of our bodies are uniquely designed to carry energy whenever it is sufficiently possible. This energy is carried as glycogen within our bodies. At any point when our blood sugar reaches levels that are too high, insulin sets off to begin the gathering all of the excess energy as glycogen so that this energy can be used at a later time. As such, any immediate and unexpected rise in blood sugar will also trigger a rise in insulin; ultimately, this will then result in more fat cells. The key idea in this is the words "immediate," or you can think of it as "sudden." A much slower increase in your level of blood sugar will generally not trigger insulin. Therefore, this will not lead to energy being stored and carried within your body as fat.

Final Summary

The very next step is to begin implementing the vast array of information resent herein. The meal plans, for instance, are an excellent way to begin gaining comfort with this approach and integrating carb cycling into your routine in a practical manner. Also, be sure to refer back to the science of carbs section which gives you detailed and valuable information about how carbs can benefit your body.

With the many demands that are so commonly associated with cars cycling and integrating a brand-new diet into your routine, you are very likely to be discouraged and nulling to try yet another diet. This may be because you did not get the goals that you thought you would garner from your other diets, or, more simply, other diets were so difficult to manage and inflicted so much harm onto your body that they proved to not be worth the time at all. However, carb cycling is different. This dietary approach allows you to uniquely tailor your diet to your needs and preferences, all the while ensuring that you are easily able to manage and calculate the results or ROI that you are receiving. This is due to the fact that carb cycling allows for constant altering and adjustments as you move through the weeks. As you do so, you will start noticing what works and what doesn't, and, most importantly, you will be keenly aware of your energy levels and how your body is responding to the different calorie levels and carbs that you consume.

Why is carb cycling so important? How will it benefit you personally form a physical and psychological perspective? These are only a few questions that are confronted and answered effectively within this text. What's more, readers will gain an abundance of knowledge pertaining to the unique benefits offered by cycling carbs and implementing carb manipulation into your dietary routine.

For athletes, whether elite or leisure, carb cycling carries many benefits that will serve to enhance your performance through boosted energy, endurance, strength and focus. Not to mention, for individuals striving to shed weight, this diet is a trusted and true strategy for losing those pesky pounds. Moreover, you are likely to have been taught that carbs are scary and should be avoided at all costs for maximized health; however, new research, such as that which is presented within this text, extinguishes these old myths, thereby providing you with the most up-to-date information about carbs and their impact on your health.

You might be a little tentative when considering the prospect of cycling carbs. Remember, this is completely normal and does not have to be an anxiety-inducing process. In fact, you should try to use your fears to motivate you to try something new with regard to your dietary routine. Indeed, you are likely to garner excellent results that will last a lifetime if committed to and implemented effectively.

Book Two

CARB CYCLING RECIPE BOOK

Simple Recipes and Meal Plans for Rapid Fat Loss, Increased Energy and Enhanced Health

Josh Falenski

Introduction

"Eat The Foods You Love – Just Cycle It!"

This book is designed to give you a quick review of the carb cycling science and how it works, then jumps right into simple, easy-to-make recipes for beginning carb-cyclers to start with. Most people never heard of "carb cycling" but are completely amazed at how fast and efficiently it works, which kind of goes against the common perception in the low-carb community; which is that carbs cause weight gain.

Like most people struggling with weight loss or health and fitness in general, I have tried almost all of the diets and weight loss techniques out there.

Every diet had a core restriction, either carbs, proteins or fat. Something was always missing. But, when I discovered "Carb Cycling", everything changed, it was the solution I was looking for.

I eventually created my own personalized daily carb cycling plan that works perfect for me. I get to enjoy the low carb foods in the first half of the day and then savor the high carb foods at night.

Not everyone will want to do a daily carb cycle, it may be that the multiple day high-low carb cycling process works better for you if you have immediate desires such as fast fat loss, or need to boost your metabolism fast.

One thing is FOR SURE, once you start carb cycling, you will finally realize that carbs are absolutely necessary or play a huge role in fat loss, energy production and a balanced hormone state, it's how and when you consume carbs that matter, as well as what type of carbs(health versus unhealthy).

Those who have been trying to lose excess pounds are probably familiar with the more popular diet fads, diet craze and diet menu plans. These diet plans' popularity stems from their promise of helping users to lose weight fast. These plans have different concepts and attacks.

Among the most recognizable are the low-carb diet plans that promise people that they will receive immediate positive results. However, some of those who tried these types of diet plans reported gaining the weight they lost right after reintroducing carbohydrates into their diets.

What is it exactly?

It's a simple diet plan that takes advantage of the benefits of reduced carbohydrate and increased carbohydrate techniques. This plan has reward days or meals, allowing you to still eat your favorites even if you're on a diet. Unlike other diet plans that restrict and completely change your eating habits, this plan does not make you feel "food-deprived". If you follow this plan, then you can still eat foods that are healthy and enjoy the foods you love, but still get rid of those excess pounds. Is it too good to be true?

The Basics

The plan allows users to go from a low-carb day to a high-carb day and a reward day each week, but it still follows some of the basics in losing weight:

- You are allowed to eat five small meals a day.

- You have to eat breakfast not later than 30 minutes after waking up. Your high-carb meal should include protein and carbohydrates.

- Succeeding meals after breakfast should have a 3-hour interval.

- The meals should include only those "approved foods".

- Consume at least 1 gallon of water or allow fluids.

How Carb Cycling Works

For you to shed off some unwanted weight, your body would need a combination of carbohydrates, proteins and fats.

- **Carbohydrates** – Carbohydrates are your body's number 1 source of fuel. You can get the carbs you need from healthy sources like fruits, vegetables, legumes and grains. Take note of the unhealthy sources of carbohydrates; some of which are cookies, cakes, doughnuts, soda, candies and processed foods. Good carbohydrates are essential for your body's ability to burn calories because they are slowly broken down by the digestive tract than those unhealthy ones. These healthy carbohydrates ensure that your body's blood sugar is kept at acceptable levels while your energy levels remain steady.

- **Proteins** – They help build and maintain muscle mass. These muscles are important in burning fat. Proteins break down more slowly than carbohydrates and fat, thus burning more calories and keep you feeling full longer.

- **Healthy fats** – These are unsaturated fats that should still be included in your diet but intake should be controlled and properly monitored. They help in the development and the proper function of your brain and eyes. They help reduce the risks of developing heart conditions and depression and prevent arthritis. They also help manage your body's energy levels and curb your appetite.

What's the principle behind alternating low-carb and high-carb days? You see, during a high-carb day, your body stocks up so that when you are on a low-carb day, you still burn unwanted fats. This actually works well with your metabolism so that your body burns more calories even during the days when you have to eat low-carb meals.

Eating more every other day and cutting down on the days in between is an effective way of intensifying the weight loss process while still efficiently maintaining your fat-burning muscles. This is a diet plan that you can use for short-term and long-term weight loss.

What Happens

Eating breakfast not later than 30 minutes after you wake up jumpstarts your body's metabolism. It also ensures that you have the fuel you need for the whole day. During your high-carb days, having your meals at three-hour intervals boosts your metabolism, provides fuel for your muscles and organs and delivers the vitamins and fibers the body needs.

On low-carb days, you burn the fat while maintaining your muscles. It also helps balance your hormones and delivers the needed vitamins and fibers to your body.

During your reward days, you reset your system so it is ready for another cycle. It helps satisfy your cravings so you don't feel deprived while losing weight. At the same time, you are rewarding yourself for your progress. It also jacks up your calorie-intake but ensures that it is limited to maintenance level. It also boosts your metabolism while developing the calorie-burning muscles.

How to Keep it Going

It would be beneficial to restart your carb-cycling engine. While this plan prevents your body from reaching a plateau, your body will eventually "understand" the process and soon your metabolism drops which will result in the slowing down of the weight loss process. In order to re-fire, you need to devote one whole week each month to eating high-carb diet only. This means that you'll be eating normally like your high-carb days. By the end of the week, your metabolism gets a big boost and it is ready to burn those calories again. This is referred to as the Slingshot technique.

<u>What are the benefits that can be derived from carb cycling?</u>

- This plan fits in any kind of lifestyle.

- You will learn the basic principles of losing weight and maintaining your ideal weight.

- You can have control over your life, not just on losing weight.

- You remain active and energy levels are always up.

- You can still eat your favorite foods.

- It helps you to build leaner and stronger muscles.

- Empowerment, physically, emotionally, mentally and spiritually.

Chapter 1: Losing Weight and the Science Behind Carb Cycling

The Science of Cycling Carbs

As a new diet, this diet is somewhat developed from the factors that undergird manipulating carbs. As such, there are still not many substantiated and controlled studies that directly investigate a carb cycling routine. In basic terms, carb cycling is a mechanism through which we try to match our body's requirement for glucose or calories.

Theoretically, this method will certainly maximize the overall benefits that carbs offer our bodies. As explained in the earlier part of this text, the benefits that carbs give our bodies are immense. While the factors that support cycling carbs certainly support its implementation, it should be viewed with some caution due to a lack of direct research about its complete effect on our health. However, this is mainly pertinent for individuals that have a history of medical concerns, especially those that have had concerns and issues related to diets that they have implemented.

The science of carb cycling converges with math, but it's rather simple math at that. On high-carb days, try to eat between 1 and 1.5 grams of carbs for every pound of your total body weight. Or make it simpler yet and set your "high-carb limit" at 200 grams on high-carb days. On low-carb days, cut this number in half. (Just remember to count only those starchy carbs; fruits and vegetables are low in carbs as well as calories and should be excluded from your "carb count.")

Here are some important things that you should keep in mind before fully implementing the carb-cycling diet into your routine for any period of time:

1. Days of High-Carb Consumption Are to Be Implemented on Intense Training Days:

Perhaps the most important thing that you should be aware of as it pertains to this to carb cycling is that you should put your highest carb consumption on days where you plan on having your most intense workout sessions. So, for instance, this means that you should be eating the most carbs on heavy workout days, or on days that involve a full body workout. This is because our bodies require carbohydrates at our most intense levels on these specific times of the week.

Moreover, consuming these prior to exercising will give your body enough fuel so that you have enough energy to push your way through the most challenging aspects of the workout. Thereafter, having carbs right after the workout will help replenish and nourish your body so that you recover fast and that your body has enough energy to have another intense workout the next day or later in the week. Specifically, this is also great for building more muscle as it will allow you to lift more weight for longer periods of time.

Because you want your carb consumption to be put to the best use possible in a manner that allows you to maximize results, along with preventing them from being converted into body fat, you have to ensure that you are timing them correctly throughout the course of the week. Planning your carb cycling, in this way, is an integral part of making sure that this method works best for you. Coupled with already having knowledge about how your body works and strategies work best for training and exercising your body, planning your intake of carbs in a strategic manner is key to getting the absolute most out of your body while training or, more generally, in your everyday life.

2. You MAY Gain Water Weight

You should also be aware of, and prepare for, possibly gaining a little bit of weight at times of implementing the high-carb day. With every carb that is consumed, your body will then hold on to 4g of water. So, when consuming 250- 350g of carbs on days of high-carb intake, this will tend to add up extremely quickly. Obviously everybody is different in how they process carbs, some bodies can metabolize carbs super-fast, and others may do so slowly at first; which may sometimes be a result of long term metabolic damage.

For people whose body composition is already leaner, they will experience this effect mostly due to water weight simply being more noticeable on their leaner body. **Not to worry, this is a completely normal process and is very common. And, thankfully, this excess water weight does not signal that your body is gaining fat. This water weight gain will certainly recede within a few days on the normal low-carb intake regimen.**

Now, it is important to be aware of whether you are someone who struggles with weight gain from a psychological perspective. If this is you, then perhaps cycling carbs is dangerous for you and you should reconsider. Indeed, temporary water weight gain tends to common accompany this dietary routine. Moreover, be prepared for this to possibly take place prior to undertaking the diet.

3. Select Carbs That Are Highest in Complex Carbohydrates or Glucose

As it pertains to selecting which food to consume when undertaking a carb cycling regimen for losing fat, you need to consider glucose. This include either sources of simple glucose (which should be consumed somewhere near the workout period where they will incidentally be absorbed much faster) or complex carbs that will be broken into glucose by your body naturally.

What should be avoided in this instance is fructose (as in high-fructose corn syrup to be specific), because this form of carb will interact differently with your body and will not have any of the positive benefits that accompany glucose.

If, for example, you consume a lot of fructose during periods of high-carb consumption, there is a high likelihood that it will be turned into fat because it will not be stored within your muscles as quickly.

4. Lower Your Fat Consumption on High-Carb Days
   Another integral consideration that you should keep in mind as you integrate a carb cycling regimen is that you need to decrease your fat intake on high-carb days. However, by lowering the overall fat intake, you will be allowing greater space for these carbs without consuming **too many** total calories.

In an ideal plan, you should try to stay within a 350-600 overall calorie limit on your days of low-carb intake in order to prevent the consumption of excess calories from being in a stalemate with your fat loss for that particular week.

5. Sustain Your Weekly Target Calorie Level for Losing Fat

As an appendage of the point above is that the overall week intake of calories should remain at a level that is needed for losing fat. For instance, when keeping your weight at 2300 calories per day, which is just slightly more than 15,400 per week, you will need to trigger an overall calorie deficit of 3500 calories per week or consume 11,900 total calories/week in order to shed one pound per week.

Standard diets require you to maintain a similar calorie level on every day of the week, this- requires you to consume 1700 calories/day. Now, consider whether you wanted to have 3 high-carb days to maximize the benefits and get the most results, you should set the calorie intake at 2400— just make sure that your weekly protein consumption remains consistent all week. As a result, because those 3 days equal nearly 7200 total calories, you will have 4700 calories that are remaining for the remaining 4 days, which is nearly 1100 calories for each. You might be able to tell that these low carb days are very low in calories; however, following high-carb days, many people will find this to be rather easy and not too much of a struggle. If, for instance, you would rather not bring you low-carb days too low on the total amount of calorie that you consume, all you really have to do is bring the overall intake of calories on high-carb days lower.

 As a result, you will get more calories for low-carb days as well. This is significant because it demonstrates that you can certainly tinker and adjust your carb cycling in a manner that works best for you. This diet regimen is not overly stringent and strenuous insofar as it limits your capacity to play around with the math. Rather, you are able to adjust the calorie and carb levels to such a degree that you reap the most benefits without having to sacrifice comfort or put too much of a strain on your body and the way that you feel.

You can probably tell that the idea of carb cycling is really about balance. Finding ways to balance your intake of carbs and calories will enhance your overall enjoyment and the benefits that you enjoy from the diet. Just be sure that your weekly intake of carbs and calories is exactly where it needs to be and that you alter and adjust accordingly. After you establish your preferences, make sure that you start to distribute all of your calories thereafter.

Simple vs. complex carbs

With the only real standout being fibers, all carbs can be absorbed directly through one's intestines and then into their blood as sugar. Moreover, this then causes blood sugar levels to rise rather rapidly. Accordingly, this form of carb will determine if the blood sugar rise is stretched over a longer period or if it is more sudden.

Simple carbs, which you should try to avoid at all costs, are primarily found in cookies, ice cream and many products that are based in flour such as pasta and dairy products. Sugar that is found within these products, along with the white flours, is broken into glucose very quickly within the digestive system. This quick breaking down means an abundant amount of glucose is then wholly absorbed through our intestines and then flows directly into our bloodstream at one time. Consequently, this leads to a spike in our blood sugar. This rise in blood sugar within our bloodstream then triggers insulin to store the remaining energy as glycogen within our fat cells—otherwise referred to as fat gain.

On the other hand, complex carbs provide energy that we all require in order to sustain our nervous system and muscles functioning devoid of excess fat— or really any fat at all. This is simply because complex carbs, which are primarily found within whole grains such as starchy food (potatoes) as well as quinoa, will take a lot longer in order to convert into glucose within our digestive system. A more prolonged breaking down results in a very slow pace of absorption into our bloodstream. In this way, a longer absorption period will mean that there will be no rise in blood sugar, resulting in no activation of insulin; therefore, there will be zero storing of energy within the fat cells in our body.

So, with all of this being considered, you should not be afraid of eating carbs! Just be sure to consume only the complex ones, rather than the far more harmful simple ones. Foods that are full of sugar— mainly those that are prepared with white flour such as pasta— are the kinds that we tend to want to eat the most. These cravings can certainly be intense. Sadly, these carbs are most harmful to us and are the main cause of gaining weight. Indeed, there is also very little to no value from a nutritional standpoint in these foods.

In contrast, complex carbs are packed with vitamins that carry great value from a nutritional perspective for our bodies. In addition to this, complex carbs can assist with losing weight because you will feel more satisfied for a long period of time. This is due to the slower breaking down within our digestive system.

The specific factors that undergird cycling carbs indicate that it is very beneficial for losing weight and even lowering your overall levels of body fat. Technically, cycling carbs all assist with sustaining a certain level of physical performance all the while offering many of the same rewards as dietary regimens that are primarily low-carbs.

Just like pretty much any diet, the primary mechanism that supports losing weight are calorie deficits— such as consuming less than what your body is able to burn off over an extended period. Now, is a diet that involves cycling cards is adopted in concert with a calorie deficit you will begin to shed weight at a relatively fast pace. However, the complexity of this integrated approach is enough to trigger confusion amongst people who are new to dieting and thus dissuade them from carrying on with the diet.

On the other hand, many individuals would prefer carb cycling's inherent flexibility. Also, this may even improve performance and results for many people, thereby allowing them to experience long-term success as well. In short, cycling your carb intake will certainly help you lose weight provided you are able to maintain a calorie deficit. Consuming ample amounts of protein is also very useful.

Among the most predominate ideas behind cycling carbs is setting a limit on carbs once your body does not require them.

Moreover, carbohydrates can be used as fuel, in the same way as gas for your vehicle, to assist your cells with performing their functions.

Consuming a lot of carbs on certain days when you are not particularly active is fairly nonsensical due to your body needing less energy— in the same way that your vehicle does not need as much gas for a short ride through town compared to a prolong trip across the country.

In fact, carbohydrates that are not burned fully result in a surplus— this can inhibit the likelihood that you will lose weight, or even result in gaining weight. On the other hand, a limit of carbohydrates to 30 grams is quite low, even on days that are not particularly active as compared to other days. 30 grams is the total amount of carbs that are found within a cup of broccoli, an apple, as well as 4 small carrots. Instead, if you are looking for a better balance, you are well advised to employ what has become more widely known as "carb matching"— this is the practice of aligning your carbohydrate consumption with all of the energy requirements that your body has. Admittedly, these will certainly vary on any given day, or periods in the day. Essentially, this method is aligned with consuming massive portions of whole carbs that are clean in order to provide more support during active hours during the day. Further, this also involves cutting your carb intake during periods of the day that are far less active. For a practical example, say you are planning to have a workout in the morning, you should eat oatmeal that is topped with some diced banana for your breakfast. However, if you are going to be in an office where you will be seated at a desk for an extended period of time, try having an avocado and veggies omelet with berries on the side. Also, as an alternative, a liquid morning diet is a great choice. Try having a protein scoop, along with some chia seed, hemp and frozen berries.

Complex carbs don't cause weight gain

A widely adopted misconception that many people tend to carry is that all carbs will cause you to gain weight and that by reducing carbs or cutting them out of your routine entirely, will boost your overall health. To fully grasp how and why this idea is flawed, you must first understand the intricate and complex ways that our bodies tend to interact with carbs— and what is the actual cause of gaining more fat onto your body.

Indeed, all of our bodies are uniquely designed to carry energy whenever it is sufficiently possible. This energy is carried as glycogen within our bodies. At any point when our blood sugar reaches levels that are too high, insulin sets off to begin the gathering all of the excess energy as glycogen so that this energy can be used at a later time. As such, any immediate and unexpected rise in blood sugar will also trigger a rise in insulin; ultimately, this will then result in more fat cells. The key idea in this is the words "immediate," or you can think of it as "sudden." A much slower increase in your level of blood sugar will generally not trigger insulin. Therefore, this will not lead to energy being stored and carried within your body as fat.

<u>Chapter 2 :</u>

Food Guidelines on Carb Cycling

Eating the right thing on specific days is vital to the success of the carb cycling program. If things did not go as planned, do not beat yourself up for it. Do not play catch up either. The program does not expect you to be perfect. It understands that there are days when things get out of your control or you simply have to have that warm bagel with creamy cream cheese that one time. There is plenty of room to adjust and get back on track. If your low-carb day turned out to be high carb, adjust your meals for the rest of the day. If you found out about it too late in the day, then take the lessons and move on with the rest of the schedule. To minimize falls, know these guidelines on eating and food choices on specific days of the carb cycling diet.

<u>Food guide on low carb days</u>

Again, breakfast is eaten within 30 minutes after getting up from bed. What to eat?

- Proteins should be palm-sized. That's about 3 ounces for women and 5 ounces of protein for men.

- Carbohydrates should be about the size of a clenched fist. That's about 1 cup for women and 1.5 cups of carbs for men.

- Non-starchy vegetables should be at least the size of 2 clenched fists. That's about 2 cups of non-starchy vegetables for women and 3 cups for men.

Breakfast is the only meal of the low-carb day that includes carbs. The rest of the day is spent eating proteins, vegetables (non-starchy), and fats.

For the rest of the day's meals and snacks (lunch, dinner and AM and PM snack), the following portions are to be observed:

- Protein portions are about the size of the palm or 3-ounce portion for women and 5-once portions for men.

- Fat portion the size of the thumb (measurement starts from the base to the tip) or 1 tablespoon for women and 2 tablespoons for men.

- Non-starchy vegetable portions at least the size of 2 clenched fists or 2 cups for women and 3 cups for men.

- Condiments, dressings and sauces are allowed but limited to no more than portions the size of the middle and index finger (measurement starts from the base to the tip).

Drinking water is important. Drink at least a gallon of water to keep good hydration.

For cravings, getting a high-fiber breakfast is an effective way of killing cravings for the rest of the day. Keep drinking water all day long to reduce cravings. Nibbling on something minty can also help. If cravings are especially strong, eat a small portion of healthy fat and follow it up with a full glass of water. Fats allowed on low-carb days include cheeses, sour cream, cream, olives and avocados, mayonnaise, creamy dressings, oils like olive oil and flaxseed oil, and a variety of seeds and nuts.

Food to avoid

Remember that breakfast is the only time for carbs on low-carb days. Also, avoid all unhealthy food like processed food, food with refined flours and refined sugars, and all sugary food. All fatty food such as French fries, artificial sweeteners, alcoholic beverages and food with high sodium contents are to be avoided as well.

Food guide on high-carb days

Calorie intake on high-carb days is 1,500 for women and 2,000 for men. To get the approximate right amount of calories, servings should be hand-sized portions. The portions are similar with the low-carb days. The difference is that carbs are eaten at every meal and snack, and no fat intake.

For breakfast (again, eat within 30 minutes of getting up) and the rest of meals and snacks (total of 3 meals and 2 snacks), portions are:

- Protein portions are about the size of the palm or 3-ounce portion for women and 5-once portions for men.

- Carbohydrates should be about the size of a clenched fist. That's about 1 cup for women and 1.5 cups of carbs for men.

- Non-starchy vegetable portions at least the size of 2 clenched fists or 2 cups for women and 3 cups for men.

- Condiments, dressings and sauces are allowed but limited to no more than portions the size of the middle and index finger (measurement starts from the base to the tip).

Food to avoid are the same- processed food, fatty food, food with refined sugars and flours, high in sodium, contains alcohol, and those with artificial sweeteners.

FOOD GUIDE FOR REWARD MEALS

Yes, you can still enjoy some great"reward food" at any of your meals, whether on low-carb or on high-carb days. That is, except for dinner because most people find it difficult to stop eating reward food at nighttime. Also, cravings tend to intensify at night, especially after eating reward food.

So what reward food can be included? Your favorite ones. If you want a sweet, honey-glazed donut for snack, go ahead. If you want ice cream, add it your lunch menu. Just make sure not to go overboard. Limit portions and do not overeat. Remember, you still have to work within your caloric requirement. The aim of the reward meal is to satisfy cravings and not to cause you to overeat. This helps to stay on track. People tend to be depressed over having to give up their favorite foods and be content with a mostly vegetable diet. And once depression sets in, cravings intensify. And once they give in, it is difficult to go back. These reward meals are tiny portions that satisfy the cravings to keep you happy and stay motivated.

In choosing your reward meal, it is vital to avoid your trigger food. Be mindful of what you eat and how you react. Trigger food are those you crave that cause you to want to eat more.

For example, eating a donut causes you to want to eat more sugary food, donut is your trigger food and you must avoid it. If eating a bag of chips causes you to crave for more - that is your trigger food. So avoid it at all cost.

Choose reward food that can satisfy your cravings and make you feel good but not because you to want more of it. If you can't determine your trigger food or you simply can't stay away from it, try substitutions. For example, if a bag of chips is your trigger food, make your reward food a bag of other salty food like pretzels. If your trigger food is chocolate, choose dark chocolates instead of the milk versions.

Chapter 3:

Breakfast Recipes
Low- Carb

Baked Eggs with Chili Oil and Spinach

Ingredients:

4 eggs

¼ teaspoon Turkish chili powder (kirmizi biber)

One pinch of paprika

10 cups spinach

3 tablespoons chopped leek

2 tablespoons chopped scallion

2/3 cup Greek yogurt, plain

1 halved garlic clove

1 teaspoon chopped oregano

2 tablespoons unsalted butter

1 teaspoon lemon juice

2 tablespoons olive oil

Salt

Procedure:

1. Combine yogurt and garlic in a mixing bowl. Season with salt and set aside.
2. Preheat the oven to 300 degrees Fahrenheit. Heat 1 tablespoon butter and oil in a frying pan. Put in the leeks and scallions and cook for 10 minutes or until they're tender.
3. Stir in the lemon juice and spinach. Add salt seasoning. Cook for about 5 minutes or until the spinach leaves are wilted.
4. Transfer the cooked spinach to a bigger pan. Create 4 wells at the center of the spinach. Break 1 egg into each well. Keep the yolks whole.
5. Bake into the preheated oven for about 10 to 15 minutes, or until the egg whites are set.
6. Heat the other 1 tablespoon of butter into the smaller frying pan. Add the Turkish spice and season with salt. Cook for about 2 minutes, and then add the oregano.
7. Remove the garlic from the mixed yogurt that was set aside earlier. Spoon the mixed yogurt over the spinach and eggs. Sprinkle with the butter and spice mixture.

Turkey Sausage and Egg White Frittata

Ingredients:

One pound turkey sausage

15 egg whites

2 bags of chopped broccoli

Procedure:

1. Cook sausage in a skillet until golden brown.
2. Mix the sausages and chopped broccoli. Season to taste.
3. Transfer the sausages and broccoli into a baking dish. Pour the egg whites over them
4. Bake at 375 degrees Fahrenheit for about 40 minutes.

Cinnamon Roll Scones

Ingredients:

For scones:

2 cups almond flour

8 drops stevia extract

2 tablespoons granulated erythritol

½ teaspoon vanilla extract

2 teaspoons baking powder

2 tablespoons heavy cream

½ teaspoon baking soda

¼ cup melted butter or coconut oil

½ teaspoon salt

1 large egg

¼ teaspoon ground cinnamon

For filling/topping:

2 tablespoons granulated erythritol

1 tablespoon brown-sugar style sweetener (optional)

2 teaspoons cinnamon

For icing:

1 oz softened cream cheese

6 drops stevia extract

1 tablespoon cream

¼ teaspoon vanilla extract

½ tablespoon softened butter

1 tablespoon powdered erythritol

Procedure:

For the filling:

1. Combine all the ingredients for the filling in a small bowl. If you do not have a brown-sugar style sweetener, you can use a teaspoon of granulated erythritol as substitute.

For the scones:

1. Heat up your oven to 325 degrees. Prepare a baking sheet and line it with parchment paper.

2. In a large bowl, combine almond flour, cinnamon, erythritol, salt, baking soda and baking powder.

3. Mix in lightly beaten egg, stevia extract, coconut oil or butter, cream and vanilla extract until the dough is formed.

4. Sprinkle the dough with half of the filling and mix lightly.

5. Put the dough in the baking sheet and shape it manually into a circle with a diameter of about 7-8 inches.

6. Sprinkle the remaining filling over the dough then cut it into 8 wedges. Make sure to separate the slices carefully and place them evenly on the baking sheet.

7. Put it in the oven and bake for about 20-25 minutes or until it becomes firm and light brown.

8. Remove from the oven. Leave it in a wire rack to cool.

For the icing:

1. Mix cream, butter and cream cheese together until it obtains a smooth consistency.

2. Add stevia extracts, powdered erythritol and vanilla into the mixture and stir until everything is combined fully.

3. Spread or pipe over your scones.

Cheesy Turkey and Peppers Quiche

Ingredients:

12 ounces seasoned turkey sausages

1 chopped green pepper

8 eggs

2 cups sliced mushrooms

1 tablespoon chipotle peppers

1/3 cup sliced green onions

¼ cup milk

¼ cup cilantro

1 cup cheddar cheese

1 tablespoon vegetable oil

Procedure:

1. Preheat oven to 350 degrees Fahrenheit. Grease a 12-muffin cup tin with oil spray.

2. Cook the turkey sausages on a skillet. Cook until well done, and then chop to little pieces.

3. Heat oil on a skillet and add mushrooms, green pepper and chipotle peppers. Cook for about 5 minutes.

4. In a mixing bowl, mix eggs, cilantro and milk. Add the turkey sausage, green pepper and mushroom mixture.

5. Put the mixture into the muffin cups. Put in the preheated oven and bake for about 20 minutes.

Lemon Muffins with Poppy Seeds

Ingredients:

56 grams coconut flour

2 scoops vanilla protein powder

1 teaspoon xanthan gum

½ cup unsweetened vanilla almond milk

¾ teaspoon baking powder

2 tablespoons freshly squeezed lemon juice

¾ teaspoon baking soda

¼ cup agave

¼ teaspoon salt

¼ cup plain non-fat Greek yogurt

1 tablespoon poppy seeds

1 teaspoon vanilla extract

1 tablespoon lemon zest

1 large egg

1 tablespoon coconut oil or melted unsalted butter

Procedure:

1. Prepare your oven by setting it up to 350 degrees. Use a non-stick cooking spray to coat 8 standard-size muffin cups lightly.

2. In a medium bowl, combine coconut flour, lemon zest, xanthan gum, poppy seeds, baking powder, salt and baking soda.

3. Put butter or coconut oil, vanilla and egg in a separate bowl and mix well. Add Greek yogurt and stir until smooth. Blend agave, almond milk, lemon juice into the mixture. Fold in protein powder.

4. Combine the two mixtures. Continue stirring until everything are mixed well. Set aside the batter for about 10 minutes to rest.

5. Put equal portions of the batter in each muffin cup. Place it in the oven for about 21-24 minutes.

6. Remove the muffin cups from the oven and insert a toothpick in the center. If it comes out clean, your muffins are done. If not, put it back in the oven and let it bake for a few more minutes.

7. Put the muffins in a pan and let them cool for about 5 minutes before setting them in a wire rack.

Turkey Omelet with Beans

Ingredients:

90 grams minced turkey

8 egg whites

1 white onion

1 mushroom

2 whole eggs

1 cup chopped red and green peppers

3 garlic cloves

1 chopped red pepper

1 tablespoon Worcestershire sauce

Procedure:

1. Heat a skillet with oil. When the skillet is hot, cook all the spices, vegetables and turkey. Sauté until the vegetables are tender.
2. Get another skillet for the omelet and heat with oil. Cook the egg mixture.
3. Wrap the egg mixture with the cooked turkey and vegetable mixture. Cook and serve hot.

Chocolate Hazelnut Waffles

Ingredients:

1 cup Hazelnut meal

¼ teaspoon stevia extract

½ cup chocolate protein powder

½ teaspoon hazelnut extract

2 tablespoon cocoa powder

3 tablespoon hazelnut oil

2 tablespoon coconut flour

1/3 cup full fat Greek yogurt

3 tablespoon granulated erythritol or sweetener

4 large eggs

Procedure:

1. Set up your oven to 200 degrees. Prepare a wire rack over a baking sheet and heat up your waffle iron to medium high.

2. Combine hazelnut meal, sweetener, protein powder, coconut flour and cocoa powder in a large bowl

3. Add eggs, stevia, yogurt, hazelnut extract and hazelnut oil into the mixture. Mix well.

4. If necessary, coat your waffle iron with grease before pouring in your batter. Make sure that each section would get about ¼ to 1/3 cup of it.

5. Close the lid and let it cook. Once the waffles are crisp brown in color, gently remove them from the iron.

6. Keep the waffles warm by placing them in the prepared baking sheets and cook the remaining batter by following the procedure above.

7. Put desired toppings as a finishing touch. You can use whipped cream, sugar free syrup, butter berries and chopped hazelnuts.

Apple Muffins

Ingredients:

2 tablespoons almond flour

2 tablespoons coconut flour

Sweetener

Cinnamon

1 chopped apple

1 Egg white

Procedure:

1. Mix all the ingredients except for the apple in a microwave-safe mixing bowl.
2. Stir well and then add the chopped apple. Put in the microwave for about 9 minutes.
3. This makes a very big muffin on a bowl. Serve hot.

Pumpkin Bagels

Ingredients:

1/3 cup sifted coconut flour

1 teaspoon sea salt

3 tablespoon golden flax meal

½ teaspoon cinnamon

3 beaten eggs

1 ¼ teaspoon pumpkin pie spice

2 tablespoon melted butter or coconut oil

1 teaspoon organic, gluten-free vanilla extract

¼ cup unsweetened almond or coconut milk

½ cup pure pumpkin puree

1 ½ tablespoons erythritol

15 drops stevia liquid

½ teaspoon baking soda

1 teaspoon apple cider vinegar

Procedure:

1. Set up your oven to 350 degrees. Apply generous amounts of oil or grease in a bagel or donut pan.

2. Mix coconut flour, sea salt, golden flax meal, cinnamon and pumpkin pie spice in a large bowl. Make sure to combine the ingredients thoroughly and set the mixture aside.

3. Place eggs, melted butter or coconut oil, pumpkin puree, erythritol, stevia extract, coconut or almond milk and vanilla extract in a separate bowl. Mix well.

4. In a pinch bowl, combine apple cider vinegar and baking soda. Add this to the egg mixture and stir well.

5. Add the resulting mixture to the coconut mixture. Continue stirring until the batter reaches a smooth consistency.

6. Pour the batter into the bagel or donut pan. Using a spatula or the back of a spoon, make sure that the batter is spread evenly. In addition, make sure that the center part of the bagel is clean by carefully wiping it with a damp paper towel.

7. Place it in the oven for about 23-25 minutes or until the top of the bagel is firm and brown in color.

8. Remove from the oven. Make sure that the bagels have completely cooled down before carefully removing them from the pan using a butter knife.

9. Apply as much cream cheese or butter as desired.

High Carb

French Toast with Strawberries

Ingredients:

4 ounces cream cheese

1 cup sliced strawberries

3 whole eggs

8 slices whole wheat bread

2 tablespoons sugar

1 cup skim milk

1 teaspoon vanilla

Strawberry jam for topping

Salt

Procedure:

1. Combine cream cheese, strawberries and sugar in a bowl.
2. In a separate mixing bowl, whisk the eggs, vanilla and milk. Season with salt.
3. Spread ¼ of the filling mixture on the slice of bread. Top with a second slice of whole wheat bread and press together.
4. Dip the bread into the egg batter.
5. Place the dipped bread into a skillet that's been greased with cooking spray.

6. Cook for about 2 minutes on each side. Top with strawberry jam and sliced strawberries.

Almond and Coconut Protein Bars

Ingredients:

2 cups rolled oats

½ cup sesame seeds

1 cup unsweetened coconut, shredded

½ cup cashews

1 cup honey

½ cup raw almonds

½ cup raw sunflower seeds

½ cup chopped raisins

1 ½ cup tahini

1 teaspoon vanilla extract

Procedure:

1. Preheat the oven to 350 degrees Fahrenheit. Grease a baking sheet with cooking spray.
2. Mix the oats, almonds, coconut, cashews, sunflower seeds, sesame seeds and chopped raisins in a mixing bowl.
3. Mix the tahini and honey in a microwaveable mixing bowl. Heat for 1 minute. Add the vanilla extract.
4. Add in the sauce to the oat mixture. Mix well.

5. Pour the mixture into the baking sheet. Mold into a rectangle. Bake in the preheated oven for 15 minutes.

Homemade Chocolate Frosted Donuts

Ingredients:

For doughnut:

1 ½ cup whole milk

5 cups all-purpose flour

1/3 cup water

1 teaspoon freshly grated nutmeg

1/3 cup unsalted butter

1 teaspoon salt

1 tablespoon honey

¼ cup sugar

4 ½ teaspoons active dry yeast

¼ cup sugar

2 large eggs

For chocolate frosting:

4 tablespoons unsalted butter

1 cup crushed kettle cooked potato chips

2 teaspoons vanilla extract

1 cup powdered sugar

1 teaspoon light corn syrup

3 oz. chopped milk chocolate

¼ cup milk

Procedure:

1. Over low heat, put water and milk in a saucepan.

2. Once warm, pour it into the bowl of the electric mixer along with butter. Stir until the butter melts.

3. Put the honey and yeast over top while giving it a quick stir. Set it aside for about 5 minutes or until the yeast becomes foamy.

4. Mix in eggs, nutmeg, salt, sugar and half of the flour into the yeast mixture. Use the paddle attachment to beat the dough.

5. Set up your machine on low speed and continue beating the dough until it gets sticky. Gradually add the remaining flour while increasing the speed to medium until the dough comes together.

6. Remove the paddle attachment and use the dough hook to beat the dough at medium speed for 5 minutes.

7. Once the dough starts to pull away from the sides of the bowl, transfer it to an oiled bowl. Cover the bowl and place it in a warm place. Your dough should rise in an hour.

8. Once it has risen, put the dough in a flat surface. Roll it out until it is 1 inch thick and use biscuit cutters to cut out the rounds and center.

9. Put the dough rounds on a baking sheet. Cover them and set aside for 30 minutes until they rise again.

10. Prepare a large pot of oil and put it over medium heat. Use a candy thermometer to monitor the temperature.

11. Once the temperature of the oil in the pot is between 365-370 degrees, drop 2-3 donuts at a time into it. Fry each side for about a minute and use a large slotted spoon to remove it from the pot.

12. Place the cooked dough on a paper towel to drain excess oil. Set it aside to cool.

13. Repeat the procedure for the remaining dough rounds. Keep in mind that the oil temperature should be maintained between 365-370 degrees at all times.

For the chocolate frosting:

1. Put a small saucepan over medium heat.

2. Add butter, milk, corn syrup and vanilla to the pan and whisk until the butter melts.

3. Decrease the heat to low before adding the chocolates.

4. Continue whisking until the mixture becomes smooth. Remove the pan from the heat and add powdered sugar. Stir well until no lumps remain.

5. Dunk the doughnuts into the glaze and sprinkle potato chips on top.

6. Set it aside for 15 minutes.

Rice Krispie Pancakes

Ingredients (pancakes):

2 cups whole wheat pastry flour

2 ¼ teaspoons baking powder

1 ½ cups of buttermilk

2 eggs

1 bag mini marshmallows

3 cups Rice Krispies

2 tablespoons melted butter

1 teaspoon vanilla extract

Salt

Ingredients (Butter Syrup):

¾ cup brown sugar

½ cup salted butter

½ cup buttermilk

1 teaspoon baking soda

1 teaspoon vanilla extract

Procedure:

1. To make the syrup, melt the butter in a pot. Slowly add the brown sugar, buttermilk, vanilla and baking soda. Blend until smooth. Boil for about 3 minutes.
2. When the syrup has thickened, remove from heat and set aside.
3. In a separate mixing bowl, blend the eggs, buttermilk, melted butter and vanilla. Combine baking powder, flour and salt.
4. Combine the wet and dry ingredients. Set aside the batter.
5. Place parchment paper on a baking dish.
6. In another pot, place 1 stick of butter and melt. Add the marshmallows. Stir for about five minutes until they melt.
7. Add ¾ cup of the melted marshmallows into the batter.
8. Add rice krispies to the remaining marshmallows in the pot. Place the mixture into the baking dish, with an even layer of rice krispie treats.
9. Heat oil on a skillet. Spoon batter into round shapes. Take a few pieces of rice krispies from the prepared mixture and place them on top of the pancakes.
10. Cook for 3 minutes, then flip and cook for another minute. Do the same for the remaining batter.

11. Drizzle the pancakes with butter syrup and a rice krispie square.

125

Fruit Scones

Ingredients:

1 cup fresh fruit (peaches, cherries, blueberries or mango, depending on preference)

1 ¾ can all-purpose flour

½ can whole wheat flour

1 cup buttermilk

1 ½ tablespoon baking powder

¾ teaspoon baking soda

½ cup sugar

1 teaspoon vanilla extract

6 tablespoons cold unsalted butter

Procedure:

1. Preheat oven to 350 degrees Fahrenheit. Place parchment paper on a round cake pan. Grease with cooking spray.
2. Mix the whole wheat flour, all-purpose flour, baking powder, baking soda and sugar in a mixing bowl. Slice the butter until they are pea sized. Coat them with flour.
3. Mix some of the buttermilk (3/4 cup) and vanilla extract in a separate mixing bowl. Add the mixture into the dry ingredients.

4. Combine the rest of the buttermilk and the fruit and
   mix well.
5. Place the mixed dough into the round cake
   pan. Slice into 8 pie-like pieces without cutting all
   the way through.
6. Place in the preheated oven and bake for 40
   minutes.

Hash Brown Casserole

Ingredients:

2 pounds frozen hash browns

2 cups grated cheddar cheese

1 can cream of chicken soup

½ cup melted butter

½ cup peeled and chopped onion

1 pint sour cream

Salt and pepper

Procedure:

1. Preheat oven to a temperature of 350 degrees F. Spray a baking dish with cooking spray.

2. Mix all the ingredients and put into the baking dish.

3. Bake in the oven for 45 minutes.

Chapter 4: Main Dishes

Low Carb

Turkey Meatballs

Ingredients:

4 pounds minced turkey

2 eggs

1 bag of cauliflower

2 tablespoons coconut flour

Chopped onions

1 can cranberry sauce

½ cup Worcestershire sauce

1 bottle chili sauce

Cajun seasoning

Salt and pepper

Procedure:

1. Cook cauliflower in the microwave. Chop the tender florets into small pieces.
2. Combine minced turkey, eggs, coconut flour, chopped onions and Worcestershire sauce. Season with Cajun seasoning, salt and pepper.

3. Mold the mixture into meatballs. Place them inside a slow cooker. Add the cauliflower.

4. Pour the cranberry sauce over the meatballs and vegetables. Pour the chili sauce over it.

5. Cook on high setting for 7 hours.

Herb Crusted Salmon

Ingredients:

For the salmon:

2 pieces 6 oz salmon fillet

1 tablespoon Dijon mustard

1 tablespoon coconut flour

1 tablespoon olive oil

2 tablespoons dried or fresh parsley

Salt and pepper

For the salad:

2 cups arugula

1 tablespoon olive oil

¼ thinly sliced red onion

1 tablespoon white wine vinegar

Lemon juice

Salt and pepper

Procedure:

1. Set up your oven to 450 degrees

2. Prepare a baking sheet and line it with foil or parchment paper. Place the salmon fillets in it.

3. Rub Dijon mustard and olive oil on your salmon fillets.

4. Combine coconut flour, salt, pepper and parsley in a small mixing bowl. Sprinkle the mixture over the fish and pat it into the fillets using your hand.

5. Place the salmon fillets in the oven. Leave it there for about 10-15 minutes or until the fish is cooked as desired.

6. Combine all of the salad ingredients. Once the fish is done, place it on top of the salad.

Cheese Enchiladas

Ingredients:

For the shells:
16 oz. bag frozen cauliflower
3 cups Monterey jack or mozzarella cheese
3 eggs

For the sauce:

½ cup chopped onion
2 cups shredded Monterey jack or pepper jack
2 large garlic cloves
2 cups shredded cheddar cheese
1 tablespoon chili powder
1 cup tomato or pizza sauce
4 tablespoons oil of choice
¼ teaspoon pepper
1 teaspoon oregano
1 teaspoon salt
2 teaspoon cumin

Procedure:

For the shells:

1. Set up your oven to 450 degrees.

2. Thaw the cauliflower and drain them. Once properly drained, dice or process them.

3. Prepare two cookie sheets and apply grease on them.

4. Combine all the ingredients for the enchilada shells. On the cookie sheets, divide the mixture into 12 6-inch round dough.

5. Bake one pan at a time. Place it in the oven for about 12-14 minutes or until the crust has turned slightly golden in color and the edges browned.

6. Remove from the oven and repeat the procedure for the second pan of shells.

7. Loosen the shells carefully from the pan once they have cooled.

For the sauce:

1. Heat up your oven to 350 degrees. Chop your garlic cloves and crush them.

2. Over medium heat, place oil in a pan and cook chili powder, garlic and onion for about 5 minutes.

3. Once the onion becomes tender, add oregano, tomato or pizza sauce, salt, cumin and pepper into the pan. Mix well until sauce is heated.

4. Combine the cheeses in a bowl.

For the enchilada:

1. Dip each shell into the sauce and place in an ungreased casserole pan. Make sure that the golden side of the shell is on top.

2. Put ¼ cup of the cheese mixture in each shell.

3. Roll the shell and place it seam-side down in the pan. Repeat the process until all of the shells have been used.

4. Pour the remaining sauce and cheese on top of the enchiladas and bake it until the cheese melts which should take about 20 minutes.

5. Remove from the oven. Put chopped fresh tomatoes, olives and shredded lettuce on top if desired.

Red Thai Curry Noodles

Ingredients:

200 grams low-carb noodles

150 grams chicken

50 grams yellow zucchini

20 ml cooking cream

5 grams red curry paste

Salt and pepper

Procedure:

1. Slice the yellow zucchini and chicken.
2. Roast the zucchini and chicken for 10 minutes. Season with salt and pepper.
3. Boil the low-carb noodles for 3 minutes in salted water.
4. Combine the cream and red curry paste to the chicken and mix well.

Honey Mustard Burgers

Ingredients:

1 lb. ground pork breakfast sausage

1 teaspoon yellow mustard

1 cup plantain chips

1 teaspoon Dijon mustard

1 egg white

1 tablespoon raw honey

3 tablespoons bacon fat

1 sliced avocado

1 minced garlic clove

½ teaspoon garlic powder

Salt and pepper

Procedure:

1. Set up your oven to 350 degrees.

2. Using a food processor, break down the plantain chips until they obtain a consistency that is similar to breadcrumbs.

3. Make 4 burger patties from the meat.

4. Whisk the egg white in a bowl until it becomes bubbly. In another bowl, place the plantain crumbs.

5. Dip each burger patty in the egg white first then to the plantain crumbs. Make sure that each patty is completely coated.

6. Sprinkle salt, garlic powder and pepper to taste.

7. Over medium heat, put bacon fat and garlic in a hot cast iron skillet. Once fragrant, sear the burgers in the pan on both sides for about 3-4 minutes. Remember that the plantain crumble should not be burned.

8. After cooking it on both sides, put the burgers in the oven for about 8-10 minutes or until they are cooked according to your preference.

9. Combine the two different kinds of mustards and honey.

10. Let the burgers rest for about 2 minutes once done. Place the honey mustard and avocado slices on top.

11. Garnish with arugula if desired.

Roasted Chicken in Lemon and Thyme

Ingredients:

One pound roasting chicken

2 lemons

6 peeled garlic cloves

6 thyme sprigs

Salt and pepper

Procedure:

1. Preheat the oven to 350 degrees Fahrenheit.
2. Sprinkle the chicken with pepper and salt.
3. Roll lemons on a work surface. Pierce the lemons about 1 inch deep using a skewer.
4. Put the lemons, garlic cloves and thyme inside the chicken cavity.
5. Truss the chicken. Season it with more salt and pepper.
6. In a large roasting pan, put the chicken with breast-side up.
7. Roast the chicken in the oven for about 2 hours or until the internal temperature is 180 degrees Fahrenheit.
8. Remove the chicken from the oven and carve.

Chili with Corn Kernels

Ingredients:

1.5 kilograms minced beef

900 grams can of diced tomatoes

1 medium can of corn kernels

2 sliced onions

400 grams salsa

½ chopped bulb of raw garlic

1 chopped red pepper

3 teaspoons chili powder

3 tablespoons olive oil

Procedure:

1. Cook the meat in a sauce pan until they turn brown.
2. Move the meat to a pot. Add olive oil, garlic and onion and cook until the onion is translucent.
3. Add the tomatoes and salsa. Simmer for 10 minutes.
4. Add the chili, pepper and corn kernels.
5. Season with chili powder and simmer for up to 50 minutes.

Soy Sauce Beef

Ingredients:

150 grams beef strips

60 grams paprika

1 chili pepper

Paprika powder

20 ml soy sauce

Pepper

Procedure:

1. Slice the paprika.
2. Roast the beef strips and paprika in a skillet for 12 minutes.
3. Add garlic. Season with salt and pepper. Combine the paprika powder.
4. Add soy sauce after 10 minutes.

High Carb

Pork and Fennel Ravioli with Shiitake Sauce

142

Ingredients:

10 ounces cubed pork tenderloin

1 ¾ cup chopped fennel

1 ½ cups chopped shiitake mushrooms

1 ½ cups chopped onion

¾ cup canned crushed tomatoes

2 minced garlic cloves

1 cup chicken broth

1/3 cup dry white wine

1 pack fresh cheese ravioli

½ teaspoon chopped rosemary

1 teaspoon fresh oregano

¼ cup grated parmesan cheese

1 tablespoon olive oil

Salt and ground black pepper

Procedure:

1. Heat oil on a frying pan. Add onions and cook until translucent.
2. Add fennel and other ingredients except for pork, tomatoes, chicken broth, rosemary and oregano. Cook for about 8 minutes.
3. Add pork and cook for a few minutes. Pour the wine and let it evaporate. Add the tomatoes and chicken broth and cook for 30 minutes.
4. Season with oregano and rosemary and cook for 5 more minutes.
5. Boil the ravioli until al dente. Drain and transfer to a platter.
6. Add the sauce and the cheese.

Mac and Cheese

Ingredients:

3 cups quinoa

1 ½ cups low-fat cheddar cheese, shredded

2/3 cup plain low-fat yogurt

1 cup whole-wheat elbow macaroni

Salt and pepper

Procedure:

1. Boil the elbow macaroni and set aside.
2. Cook the quinoa and set aside.
3. Mix the quinoa and macaroni.
4. Mix in the cheese and yogurt. Season with salt and pepper.
5. Top with cheese.

Vegetable and Polenta Casserole

Ingredients:

1 sliced eggplant

2 cups polenta

1 ½ cups marinara sauce

2 sliced yellow squash

4 Portobello mushrooms

1 bunch of asparagus

½ cup crumbled goat cheese

8 cups water

¼ cup chopped basil

2 tablespoons olive oil

Salt

Procedure:

1. Preheat the grill. Brush all the vegetables – mushrooms, asparagus, squash and eggplant with oil.
2. Put the vegetables on the grill and cook for about 4 minutes. The eggplant will have to be cooked for about 6 minutes.
3. Remove the vegetables and slice the mushroom into strips.
4. In a sauce pan, mix salt and water and boil.

5. Add in the polenta. Cook and stir for about 30 minutes.

6. Preheat the oven for 375 degrees Fahrenheit.

7. Place ½ cup of marinara sauce on the bottom of a baking dish. Add ½ of the cooked polenta. Layer the grilled vegetables. Spread the rest of the polenta on top. Top with the remaining marinara sauce.

8. Sprinkle with basil and cheese.

9. Cover the layered mixture with foil and bake for 30 minutes.

Turkey-Feta Meatballs on Penne

Ingredients:

1 pound penne

1 ½ pounds minced turkey

¾ cup crumbled feta cheese

½ cup crumbled saltines

8 garlic cloves

1 egg

4 slices chopped prosciutto

1 tablespoon tomato paste

½ teaspoon dried oregano

1 cup red wine

2 cans crushed tomatoes

7 cups water

¼ cup olive oil

Salt

Procedure:

1. Heat oil in a large frying pan. Add the garlic cloves. Toast for 5 minutes. Remove, then smash and mince.

2. In a mixing bowl, break up the turkey, then add the feta, oregano and saltines. Mix well.

3. Combine the egg, toasted garlic and tomato paste in another bowl. Add the meat mixture and mix well. Mold them into meatballs.

4. Heat oil in a pot. Add the meatballs. Transfer to a serving platter.

5. Place the minced garlic and prosciutto to the pot. Cook for 1 minute. Mix in the wine, tomatoes and water. Simmer.

6. Add the meatballs and cook for 15 minutes.

7. Mix in the remaining 6 cups of water to the pot. Season with salt and simmer.

8. Add the penne and cook until it is al dente. Simmer and adjust the seasonings.

9. Garnish with feta cheese before serving.

Pitas with Chicken and Sun-Dried Tomato

Ingredients:

4 whole wheat pitas, sliced in half

8 ounces rotisserie chicken

2 garlic cloves

¼ cup walnuts

1 ½ cup arugula

1 sliced avocado

¼ cup fresh mint

1 cup sliced roasted bell peppers

10 sun-dried tomatoes in oil

2 tablespoons oregano

2 tablespoons warm water

Cayenne pepper and salt

Procedure:

1. Soak the sun-dried tomatoes in warm water for about 30 minutes.
2. Mix the soaked sun-dried tomatoes, garlic, mint, oregano, red peppers, water and walnuts in a food processor. Season with salt and cayenne pepper.
3. Process until the mixture is smooth.

4. Put 1 tablespoon of the tomato spread in each
   pita. Stuff the pita with chicken, avocado, arugula
   and some of the red peppers.

Chapter 5:

Sides Dish

Low-Carb

Chicken Salad

Ingredients:

150 grams chicken

Leafy greens

1 egg

40 grams chickpeas or garbanzo beans

10 grams mustard

15 ml vinegar

Curry powder

10 ml olive oil

Salt and pepper

Procedure:

1. To prepare the mustard marinade, place vinegar, olive oil and mustard into a mixing bowl. Mix well. Season with salt and pepper.
2. Slice chicken and roast for 12 minutes on a roasting pan.
3. Season the chicken with curry powder and salt and pepper.

4. Wash the leafy greens and arrange on a platter. Add the roasted chicken, chickpeas or garbanzo beans and egg.
5. Drizzle the mustard marinade and add fresh dill.

No-Potato Salad

Ingredients:

2 heads cauliflower

1 teaspoon yellow mustard

1 dozen hard-boiled eggs

1 ½ cup mayonnaise

½ medium-sized red onion

6-8 finely diced celery stalks

Diced dill pickles

Black pepper

Procedure:

1. Cut cauliflower into large florets

2. Steam the florets for about 7-10 minutes or until tender. Keep in mind that the cauliflower should be soft but not mushy.

3. After rinsing in cold water, drain the steamed cauliflower and use paper towel to pat them dry.

4. In a large mixing bowl, crumble the cauliflower and add all the remaining ingredients. Mix well.

Beef Carpaccio with Lemon Dressing

Ingredients:

200 grams beef Carpaccio

10 ml olive oil

20 grams parmesan cheese

10 ml lemon juice

Pepper

Procedure:

1. Combine olive oil and lemon. Add them to the Carpaccio beef.
2. Add pepper and parmesan cheese.

Tuna Salad, Italian-Style

Ingredients:

150 grams tuna

30 grams olives

80 grams leafy greens

10 ml vinegar

5 ml olive oil

Garlic powder

Salt and pepper

Procedure:

1. Cut the leafy greens.
2. Combine with tuna and olives.
3. In a mixing bowl, stir in vinegar and olive oil. Add garlic powder. Season with salt and pepper.
4. Mix the prepared dressing with the leafy greens, tuna and olives.

Shrimp and Avocado Salad

Ingredients:

For the marinade/dressing:

3 tablespoons lime juice

1/8 teaspoon fresh cracked pepper

 2 tablespoons extra virgin olive oil

1/2 cup of chopped fresh cilantro

Salt

For the salad:

Cilantro dressing

4 cups baby greens or lettuce

1 lb. cooked shrimp

2 ripe avocados

Procedure:

1. Put all marinade ingredients in a bowl and mix well.

2. Remove the vein and tail of the shrimp and let it soak in the marinade. Make sure to coat the shrimp fully with it.

3. Cover the bowl and put it in the refrigerator for at least an hour. You may want to let the shrimp soak longer in the marinade to enhance the flavor.

4. Wash the lettuce. You can choose to pat them dry using a paper towel or just leave them sitting in a colander. Distribute among plates equally.

5. Slice the avocado into bite-sized portions and spread over the lettuce.

6. Put the marinated shrimp on top and drizzle with leftover dressing.

BEAT Salad

Ingredients:

1 ripe avocado

2 boiled eggs

1 medium-sized tomato

1 lemon wedge

2-4 pieces of cooked pieces

Salt and Pepper

Mayonnaise (optional)

Procedure:

1. Chop the avocado, eggs and tomato into chunks. Slice the bacon into tiny bits and squeeze the lemon wedge to get the juice.

2. Combine all ingredients carefully. Only a portion of the egg and avocado should be reduced to mush.

3. Add a spoonful of mayonnaise if desired.

Curried Chicken Salad with Egg and Avocado

Ingredients:

150 grams sliced chicken

1 chopped egg

30 grams chopped avocado

35 grams chopped onion

Leafy greens (any variety)

5 ml olive oil

Vinegar

Curry powder

Salt and pepper

Procedure:

1. Roast the sliced chicken pieces in medium heat for 15 minutes. Season with salt, pepper and curry powder.
2. Mix the avocado, egg and onion and combine with the leafy greens. Drizzle olive oil and vinegar.
3. Add the curry chicken over the salad.

Tuna Salad with Avocado and Tomato

Ingredients:

150 grams fresh tuna steak

1 sliced avocado

2 chopped tomatoes

1 onion

150 grams cooked lima beans

8 asparagus tips

1 tablespoon lemon juice

2 tablespoons olive oil

Salt and pepper

Procedure:

1. Brush the tuna steak with olive oil and fry for about 3 minutes on each side.
2. Steam the asparagus tips until tender.
3. Place the beans on a platter with the chopped tomatoes, onion and sliced avocado.
4. In a mixing bowl, thoroughly mix the olive oil and lemon juice to make a dressing. Season to taste with salt and pepper.
5. Pour the dressing over the vegetable and bean salad.
6. Slice the cooked tuna and combine with the vegetables.

7. Drizzle the remaining dressing over the tuna, beans
    and vegetables.

Enchilada Chicken Salad

Ingredients:

1 small head of hearts of romaine

½ avocado

1-2 cups cold enchilada chicken

1 peeled mango

Salt and Pepper

Procedure:

1. Shred and chop the romaine.

2. Put the leftover enchilada chicken above it.

3. Dice the mango and avocado. Place the fruits on top of the chicken meat.

Chef Salad in Ham Cups

Ingredients:

2 thin slices of ham

Shredded lettuce

Chopped tomatoes

Chopped hard-boiled egg

Shredded cheddar cheese

Procedure:

1. Set up your oven to 350 degrees.

2. On a cookie sheet, put a muffin pan or a couple of inverted custard cups.

3. Put the ham slices over the custard cup or muffin pan.

4. Place a second custard cup over the ham slices.

5. Remove any excess amount of ham from the bottom but make sure to leave about 1.2 inch or so.

6. Put it in the oven for about 20 minutes

7. After carefully removing from the oven, let the ham cups cool in a rack.

8. Remove the top custard cup and set it aside for a few minutes. Once the ham cup is cool enough,

remove it from the second custard cup or muffin pan.

9. Fill each cup with lettuce, tomato, egg and cheese.

High Carb

Clam Chowder

Ingredients:

2 diced celery stalks

1 diced onion

3 cubed russet potatoes

1 can fat-free evaporated milk

2 teaspoons minced garlic

28 ounces can of clams

18 ounces bottle of clam juice

1 tablespoon olive oil

Procedure:

1. Sauté the onions and celery in olive oil in a frying pan.
2. Transfer the sautéed vegetables into the slow cooker. Mix in the other ingredients except for the milk.
3. Cook on high setting for three hours.
4. Add the milk during the last hour. Season with pepper and salt.

Mixed Vegetable Minestrone

Ingredients:

1 can diced tomatoes with juice

1 can rinsed and drained chickpeas or garbanzo beans

2 cups baby kale

1 chopped carrot

3 chopped celery ribs

½ chopped sweet onion

3 chopped garlic cloves

A handful of shredded fresh basil

4 cups vegetable broth

Salt and black pepper

Procedure:

1. Mix all ingredients except for kale and seasoning in a sauce pan. Boil and simmer for 40 minutes.
2. Add the kale and cook for 10 minutes. Put fresh basil and season with salt and pepper.

Ham and Corn with Scalloped Potatoes

Ingredients:

6 cups cubed potatoes

1 ½ cups cooked ham, cubed

2 tablespoons all-purpose flour

¼ cup of green bell pepper, chopped

1 can cheddar cheese soup

½ cup milk

2 teaspoons minced onion

1 can whole kernel sweet corn, drained

Procedure:

1. In a slow cooker, put ham, potatoes, corn, onion and bell pepper. Mix well.
2. In a separate mixing bowl, mix cheese soup, flour and milk. Whisk until smooth.
3. Combine the potato mixture and soup mixture. Mix well.
4. Cook on slow cooker for 9 hours.

Baked Russet Potato Soup

Ingredients:

1 chicken bouillon

¼ cup butter

2 stalks green onions, chopped

2 garlic cloves

1 quart milk

¼ cup flour

15 peeled and cubed russet potatoes

Salt and pepper

Optional: cheese and bacon

Procedure:

1. Boil the potatoes in a pot for about 20 minutes.
2. Drain the potatoes. Reserve 4 cups of the water.
3. In a different pot, mix in the bouillon and butter. Add green onions, garlic and flour. Mix well until smooth.
4. Stir in the milk and potato water. Mix until thick, like a white sauce.
5. Add the boiled potatoes.
6. Top with cheese, bacon pieces and green onions

Bruschetta with Tomato and Basil

Ingredients:

½ whole-grain baguette, sliced diagonally

2 minced garlic cloves

1 tablespoon chopped parsley

2 tablespoons chopped basil

3 diced tomatoes

½ cup diced fennel

2 teaspoons balsamic vinegar

1 teaspoon olive oil

Black pepper

Procedure:

1. Toast the sliced baguette in the oven at 400 degrees Fahrenheit.
2. Combine all the other ingredients.
3. Spoon the mixture over the baguette and serve.

Conclusions

The very next step is to begin implementing the vast array of information resent herein. The meal plans, for instance, are an excellent way to begin gaining comfort with this approach and integrating carb cycling into your routine in a practical manner. Also, be sure to refer back to the science of carbs section which gives you detailed and valuable information about how carbs can benefit your body.

With the many demands that are so commonly associated with cars cycling and integrating a brand-new diet into your routine, you are very likely to be discouraged and nulling to try yet another diet.

This may be because you did not get the goals that you thought you would garner from your other diets, or, more simply, other diets were so difficult to manage and inflicted so much harm onto your body that they proved to not be worth the time at all. However, carb cycling is different.

This dietary approach allows you to uniquely tailor your diet to your needs and preferences, all the while ensuring that you are easily able to manage and calculate the results or ROI that you are receiving. This is due to the fact that carb cycling allows for constant altering and adjustments as you move through the weeks. As you do so, you will start noticing what works and what doesn't, and, most importantly, you will be keenly aware of your energy levels and how your body is responding to the different calorie levels and carbs that you consume.

Why is carb cycling so important? How will it benefit you personally form a physical and psychological perspective? These are only a few questions that are confronted and answered effectively within this text. What's more, readers will gain an abundance of knowledge pertaining to the unique benefits offered by cycling carbs and implementing carb manipulation into your dietary routine.

For athletes, whether elite or leisure, carb cycling carries many benefits that will serve to enhance your performance through boosted energy, endurance, strength and focus. Not to mention, for individuals striving to shed weight, this diet is a trusted and true strategy for losing those pesky pounds.

Moreover, you are likely to have been taught that carbs are scary and should be avoided at all costs for maximized health; however, new research, such as that which is presented within this text, extinguishes these old myths, thereby providing you with the most up-to-date information about carbs and their impact on your health.

You might be a little tentative when considering the prospect of cycling carbs. Remember, this is completely normal and does not have to be an anxiety-inducing process. In fact, you should try to use your fears to motivate you to try something new with regard to your dietary routine.

Indeed, you are likely to realize excellent results that will last a lifetime you are committed to this and implement it effectively, like anything else in life.

www.ingramcontent.com/pod-product-compliance
Lightning Source LLC
Chambersburg PA
CBHW031115250726
48655CB00004B/1721